COCKT/

COCKTAIL

by

VINCE LICATA AND PING CHONG

A play about the life and HIV drug development work of
Dr. Krisana Kraisintu

SILKWORM BOOKS

ISBN 978-974-9511-68-8

For production information, please contact:
Ping Chong & Company
47 Great Jones St.
New York, NY 10012
Tel: 212-529-1557
Email: info@pingchong.org

Published in 2009 by
Silkworm Books
6 Sukkasem Road, T. Suthep
Chiang Mai 50200 Thailand
info@silkwormbooks.com
http://www. silkwormbooks.com

All photographs courtesy of Dr. Krisana Kraisintu
Cover photograph: Pandit Watanakasivish
Cover design: Trasvin Jittidecharak
Typeset in ScalaSans 10 pt. by Silk Type
Printed and bound in Thailand by O.S. Printing House, Bangkok

5 4 3 2 1

CONTENTS

FOREWORD

Cocktail is the story of Krisana Kraisintu, whose crusade has been to make HIV/AIDS drug treatments accessible in HIV-ravaged third-world countries around the world. Starting in her native Thailand, this pharmaceutical chemist defied first-world patents and restrictions to create an inexpensive fixed-dose combination pill and has been instrumental in creating manufacturing facilities throughout Africa and the Far East. Pitted against corporate greed and political corruption, Kraisintu continues to struggle for the resources needed to stem the tide of the HIV/AIDS epidemic throughout impoverished third-world nations.

But this play is not a documentary per se. Vince LiCata is an associate professor in the departments of Biological Sciences and Chemistry whose research is directly related to anti-HIV drugs. He's also an accomplished playwright whose unique interests have drawn him into reflections on the common ground that exists in the processes and procedures that are used to "make" both science and art. As such, *Cocktail* is tapping into a growing tradition in contemporary theater. From Stoppard's *Hapgood* and *Arcadia* to Michael Frayn's *Copenhagen*, and to Kirsten Sheperd-Barr's 2006 study, *Science on Stage*, it is becoming increasingly apparent that the sciences/arts intersection is a rich vein ready to be tapped.

However, having the internationally renown Ping Chong onboard as coauthor and director places *Cocktail* on new ground in this developing

---

William W. Demastes is Professor of English at Louisiana State University at Baton Rouge. This is a review of a performance of *Cocktail*, directed by Ping Chong, at Swine Palace Theater, Baton Rouge, LA, May 6, 2007.

genre. For dramatic purposes, Chong and LiCata must manipulate the "story" of the rise of HIV/AIDS in the third world and Kraisintu's contributions to stemming the tide. Making good theater, like making good science, requires creative input rather than merely pedestrian or journalistic technical skills. The result of this collaboration in the theater is far more than the sum of its parts. Ping Chong visited LiCata's laboratory, listening to LiCata's thoughts on the nature of the molecular universe that LiCata and Kraisintu enter through their work. LiCata absorbed Chong's metaphors concerning the precision and aesthetic efficiency of Japanese tea ceremonies, a physical choreography he found organically analogous to the hands-on work of science. The result, on the stage, is a narrative that is less "told" than it is experienced. Images abound and impressions remain imprinted in the memory long after leaving the theater.

Discovering ways to effectively combine three anti-HIV regimens into a single treatment, Kraisintu's lab work was itself something of an artistic enterprise. On stage, *Cocktail* draws together a variety of inspirations, random influences, and coincidences into an imagistic dance that replicates the non- or anti-linear path(s) to true discovery. Science is not the pre-Kuhnian vision of linear progress toward a targeted goal. It involves serendipity as much as it does hard work over a piece of exotic lab equipment. And so the story of Kraisintu is a journey that has its beginning, middle, and end. But the journey sometimes goes far afield—literally, for example, into jungles riddled by civil war—as it struggles to reach its final destination. Good guys and bad guys become indistinguishable, and dead ends convert to opportunities at the most unexpected of times.

Traveling with high-speed intensity from Asia to North America, Europe, and Africa, *Cocktail* generates a full, almost visceral, recognition that our planet is shrinking. A play like *Cocktail* takes other channels than our politicians and world leaders in their efforts to mobilize a sometimes apathetic populace to respond to crises thousands of miles from home. *Cocktail* reminds us that we're all neighbors and it succeeds at making us truly *feel* that point.

Introduction

Tamara Loos

The "luxurious" Impala Shuttle may set the world's record for advertising misnomers. No one would, at first glance, imagine likening it to the sleek African antelope after which it is named, nor does it remind one of anything remotely luxurious, jerking along the pitted road that runs 255 kilometers between Nairobi and Arusha in East Africa. A small child could swim in one of the potholes. I was on my first trip to Africa. My older brother had dared me to climb Mt. Kilimanjaro with him for our birthdays, both in January, and for reasons established in childhood, I was honor-bound to meet his challenge. By mid-January 2007 we found ourselves bouncing toward Arusha in Tanzania, sitting in the only two open seats at the very back of the bus and relieved that they let us board at the last minute. We had not made a single reservation. For anything.

The bus had already filled with the most startling array of colors, both in the *kanga* and *kitenge* cotton sarongs wrapped around some of the female passengers, and in the ethnic diversity of my fellow riders. I sat next to a Muslim Gujarati and his adult son, whose family had lived in Tanzania for generations. They exchanged greetings with a Muslim woman who hailed from one of the many tribes that comprise the population of Tanzania. Riveting my attention by turns was the countryside jolting by, which offered

Tamara Loos is an associate professor of Southeast Asian history at Cornell University. She would like to thank the following people for their part in helping her write this introduction: Tom Loos, James Loos, Coeli Barry, Sandy Crandall, Trasvin Jittidecharak, Patricia "Trish" Suchy, Ping Chong, and most of all to Vince LiCata for his feedback and advice, and to Achara Eksaengsri and Krisana Kraisintu, who graciously invited her into their lives.

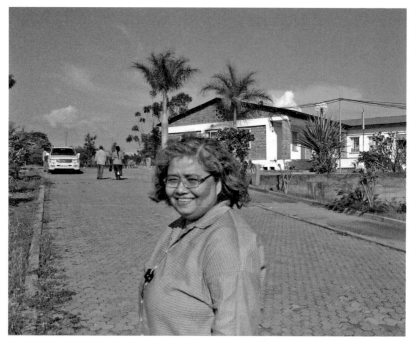

Dr. Krisana at St. Camillus Hospital in Karungu, Kenya, September 2008.

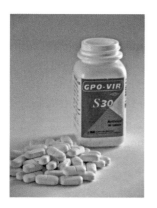 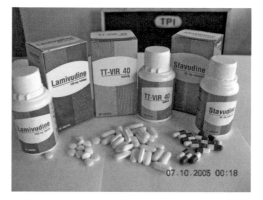

Left, GPO-VIR. Right, TT-VIR 40, a fixed-dose combination drug for HIV/ AIDS treatment manufactured at Tanzania Pharmaceutical Industries (TPI), Tanzania, October 2005.

views of enormous malicious-looking ant-hills with gaping mouths ready at any moment to emit a scourge, as well as familiar, yet oddly incongruous Coca Cola advertisements adorning the flimsy corrugated rooftops of restaurants with names like the Oysterbay Bar and the Flamingo.

The range of languages that babbled along with the scenery made it an auditory experience that placed me as an outsider, given that I know no Swahili, Arabic, Gogo, or other language, besides English, spoken in East Africa. Because I am a historian of Thailand I do, however, speak Thai, which is why I felt an urgent sense of relief and belonging when I heard someone up a few rows, sitting in a coveted window seat, speaking central Thai. She appeared to be issuing commands to some imaginary underling as I could see no other passenger engaged in a conversation with her. The sheer oddity of traveling on the Impala Shuttle through East Africa with my older brother on one side, a Muslim of South Asian descent on the other, and a woman speaking Thai somewhere in the crowd of mostly East Africans in front of me became one of those frozen moments of time: it was too strange and personal to be coincidental, and I felt that my life was about to change.

"Are you from Bangkok?" I asked politely in Thai, projecting my voice expectantly towards the stranger. Her back towards me, she twisted her neck so she faced me and pulled her glasses warily down over her nose to get a better look at who had been eavesdropping on the animated conversation she was having on her Bluetooth. I surprised her too, speaking Thai with an eager smile, but dressed in the grating Western white tourist uniform of a wicking T-shirt and khaki Northface pants that zip off at the knee. I couldn't tell if she was pleased or annoyed.

In retrospect, I like to think her face registered intrigued surprise. That ambiguous moment began what has become a relationship of unequivocal respect and admiration for Dr. Krisana Kraisintu (her family name is pronounced "grai-sin"), a pharmaceutical miracle worker whose name deserves to be known and recognized throughout the world. Dr. Krisana, a Thai national, has single-handedly saved tens of thousands of lives in Thailand,

Africa, and elsewhere by formulating and manufacturing affordable generic drugs to treat HIV/AIDS, malaria, and other maladies that strike the poor in particular. In Thailand in 1995, after six long months of grueling, solitary toil with toxic raw materials in a windowless storage room-turned-lab, Dr. Krisana formulated the generic version of AZT, an antiretroviral (ARV). AZT is not only used to treat HIV generally but also is given to pregnant women infected with the virus because it reduces their chances of passing on HIV to their children. Dr. Krisana also was the first to create the generic "cocktail," or fixed-dose combination, that combines three generic ARVs in one pill.[1] Her generics, which cost less than a dollar a day, are many times less expensive than their branded counterparts. People with AIDS take the generic "cocktail" pill, called GPO-VIR, twice a day instead of taking six different pills, ensuring greater compliance to the previously onerous drug regime required to treat the virus. Her fixed-dose combination of antiretrovirals has become the industry standard for lesser developed countries.

Perhaps more remarkable for its long-term consequences is her audacious and unwavering conviction that "teaching people how to fish is better than giving them fish." Dr. Krisana provides gratis her generic drug formulas to the African countries with which she works, trains Africans how to make the drugs and maintain quality control, and ensures that the drugs are sold at affordable prices for local consumption. She, in short, transfers technological know-how to the poorest African countries—including the Democratic Republic of Congo, Tanzania, Mali, and Liberia, among others—in order to break the cycle of dependency of lesser developed countries on the wealthier countries and multinational pharmaceutical companies. And there she was

---

1. Dr. David Ho created the "cocktail," which refers to the concept of using three drugs at one time, in 1995. Dr. Krisana was the first to combine three drugs into a single pill, which is called a fixed-dose combination or FDC. I am grateful to Dr. Vince LiCata for explaining this and other important details regarding antiretrovirals and HIV/AIDS drug therapies.

sitting right in front of me on the bus to our hotel in Arusha, Tanzania, one of her homes away from home.[2]

Since then we have met frequently. In Baton Rouge, Louisiana, I had the unique pleasure of observing Dr. Krisana watch the rousing, inspirational play, *Cocktail*, cowritten by director Ping Chong and molecular biology professor Vince LiCata. Dr. Krisana invited me to the play, which is about her mission to create generic life-saving medicines, because she had originally asked me to write her biography based on her Thai language diaries that she keeps while in Africa. Once I watched the play I felt elated by the dramatic and yet reliable representation of her life, but also obsolete because LiCata and Ping had told her tale so well. In fact, Dr. Krisana sat in the audience nearly every night for the week she visited Baton Rouge as LSU's Chancellor's Distinguished Lecturer, and each time surprised LiCata and Chong by saying to the rapt audience, "This is exactly what my life was like." Although the play cannot represent the entire truth of her experience as a youth, at the GPO, and in Africa, it accurately reflects the feelings she connects to certain times, places, and the difficult decisions she had to make in her short fifty-six years.

Split into two parts, the first half of the play covers her achievements in Thailand between 1983 and 2002, when Dr. Krisana worked for Thailand's Government Pharmaceutical Organization (GPO). By 1989 she had risen to

---

2. There are several excellent interviews with Dr. Krisana published and available in Thai and English. This introduction made use of these published interviews, my own interviews with her, and her first autobiography. The two most complete and compelling interviews are: "Raeron chiwit thi rai chutmai plaithang" (Gypsy Life with No Future), *Sakulthai* 2803 (July 8, 2008), http://www.krisana.org (accessed September 4, 2008); and Ashok Mahadevan, "Asian of the Year 2008: The Medicine Maker," *Reader's Digest* (January 2008), 28–35. Her first autobiography is called *Phesachakon yipsi* (Gypsy Pharmacist) (Bangkok: Lips Pub. Co. Ltd., 2007). National Public Radio is among the few national U.S. news organizations that have interviewed Dr. Krisana. See Richard Knox, "A Thai Woman's Fight for AIDS Drugs for All," *Morning Edition*, National Public Radio, July 12, 2004, http://www.npr.org/templates/story/story.php?storyId=3301021 (accessed October 3, 2008).

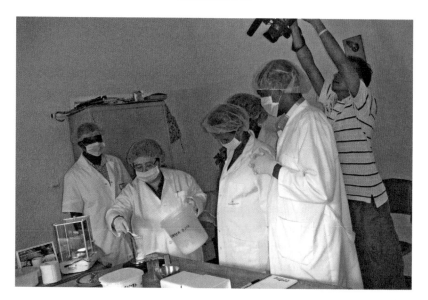

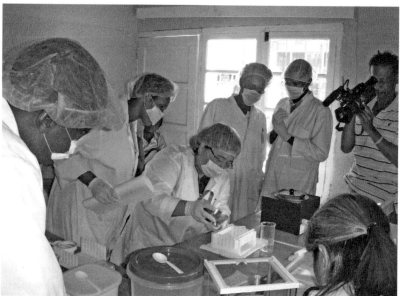

Artesunate suppositories (for malaria treatment in pediatric patients) at Centre Medical Dohero, Bujumbura, Burundi, September 2008.

the position of director of the Research and Development Institute which she grew from one staff member (herself) to over seventy, and which she dedicated to the manufacturing of new drugs never produced before in Thailand. By the time she left the GPO in 2002, she had shepherded the manufacturing of over one hundred new kinds of drugs, from generic anti-malarials and antiretrovirals, to common acetaminophen and delicious syrups to treat a variety of illnesses that afflict children. The GPO was generating a profit for the first time and, thanks to Dr. Krisana, had checked Thailand's HIV/AIDS epidemic. The second half of the play focuses on her experiences in the war-torn Democratic Republic of Congo, where Dr. Krisana began working in 2002. There she cemented her new life mission to transfer drug manufacturing technology to lesser developed African nations.

Cocktail begins with flashbacks to Dr. Krisana's childhood when her maternal grandmother, a woman who became a Buddhist nun later in her life, heavily influenced her moral mission. These scenes, sculpted into art by Ping Chong's visual designs and auditory techniques, were written on the basis of interviews she gave with Chong and LiCata. They touched Dr. Krisana most profoundly. The silhouette of young Krisana kneeling at her grandmother's side evokes a sense of the mystical and mythical, much like the lessons Krisana learned from her grandmother's example. Her grandmother is credited with freeing her slaves long before Krisana's birth, after which time she had taken the vows of a Buddhist nun at a local temple on Samui Island. At a young age Krisana witnessed her grandmother's compassionate acts of generosity for those less fortunate, especially for farmers toiling on Samui's soil. Her grandmother also pushed Krisana to persevere against all odds, as she intones in the play, "never give up." These principles guide Dr. Krisana's actions in Africa today, where obstacles are the norm.

Dr. Krisana's grandmother may have shaped her moral mission, but other family members channeled her energies into the field of medicine.[3]

---

3. The information about Dr. Krisana's childhood and family stems from multiple interviews conducted with her in 2007 and 2008.

Dr. Krisana comes from a long line of medical practitioners. Her maternal grandfather, who hails from a political family (Wichaidit) now associated with the Democratic Party in the south, practiced Thai traditional medicine in addition to serving as the governor of Samui and owning a printing company. Her father, a quiet and resourceful man whose own father raised elephants and grew rice in Surat Thani, became a doctor, thanks to the Thai government, which subsidized his education. He met Dr. Krisana's mother at a health center on Samui where she worked as a nurse. Her mother's family welcomed the marriage despite the differences in their class backgrounds because he devoted his life to medicine. The couple welcomed Krisana into the world in February 1952, and then her brother a few years later.

Krisana grew up in her maternal grandparents' home, which was large enough to accommodate three families: Krisana's natal family as well as the families of two of her mother's sisters. As a child, young Krisana witnessed pain, illness, and medical miracles in her home, the back of which supported a maternity clinic where Krisana's mother helped the women of Samui deliver babies and recuperate. Her father worked for the Ministry of Public Health and charged very little for his services, which were paid in kind more often than not. The strong silent type, her father spoke infrequently but sagaciously. From her father, who passed away years ago from cancer, Krisana inherited resourcefulness: she, like him, can fix any machine, a skill that comes in handy in Africa, where pharmaceutical equipment breaks down frequently and repairs must be done on site.

Her grandmother's emphasis on simplicity and detachment to the wealth she inherited, and her parents' work with the less affluent of Samui, shaped Krisana's moral worldview and kept her grounded literally in the blood and sweat that stained the lives of those around her. Sent to boarding school at the exclusive Rajini School in Bangkok, she quickly developed the skill of mixing with high society while staying firmly grounded in principles she learned on Samui. For a change in scenery, the restless Krisana decided to pursue a degree in pharmacy at Chiang Mai University in northern Thailand, which she completed in 1975. Soon thereafter she journeyed to Scotland

and England where she perfected her English by studying Shakespeare and literature at Cambridge and other schools before buckling down to study for a master's in pharmaceutical analysis from Strathclyde University in Scotland, and for a Ph.D. in pharmaceutical chemistry from the University of Bath in England, which she received in 1981. She returned to southern Thailand where she taught in the pharmaceutical chemistry department at the Prince of Songkla University, but Dr. Krisana felt she could make a much bigger difference if she worked with the Government Pharmaceutical Office, which manufactures medicines for Thailand's population. With her father's assistance, Dr. Krisana secured a position in 1983 at the GPO where her drive and skills were rewarded with the appointment as Director of the Research and Development Institute in 1989.

There she met a colleague who would become her most committed supporter and friend, Achara Eksaengsri. Achara appears in the play as Dr. Krisana's "go-to" girl, part secretary and part scientist. She too has a background in pharmaceutical science. She met Dr. Krisana in the mid-1980s at the GPO, where Dr. Krisana stood out in Achara's mind because she, unlike all the other women working in the GPO, was taciturn and focused on the public health issues confronting Thailand. They worked so well together that when the director of the GPO appointed Dr. Krisana as head of the research and development division, Dr. Krisana asked Achara to join her as chief of the Information Unit. With Dr. Krisana's encouragement, Achara, who had no previous knowledge of information technology or intellectual property rights, became one of Thailand's patent experts. In 2008 she became the GPO's new director of the Research and Development Institute. Her devotion to Dr. Krisana's cause and Dr. Krisana's reliance on Achara's organizational and logistical skills sustain their enduring friendship, as the play demonstrates.

Cocktail picks up on the thread of Dr. Krisana's life at the GPO, where she encountered people in power, like the derisive politician portrayed in the play who condemned all individuals who contracted HIV/AIDS—including fetuses in the womb—as deserving to die. Her three-hour argument with

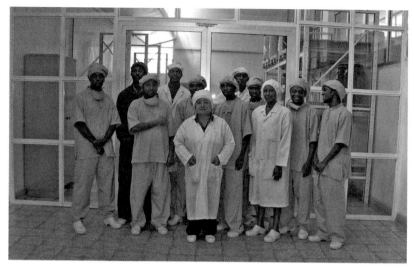

Dr. Krisana and her team at the antiretroviral production unit at TPI, Tanzania, October 8, 2005.

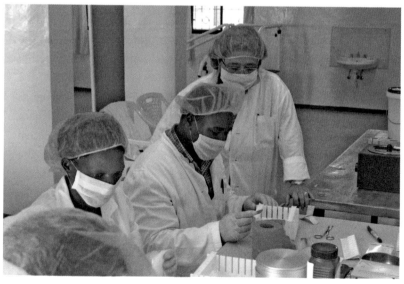

Artesunate suppositories (for malaria treatment in pediatric patients) at St. Camillus Hospital in Karungu, Kenya, September 2008.

the politician, then head of one of Thailand's most important and powerful parties, is not fictional. It catalyzed Dr. Krisana to not only quit the party, but to commit to creating a drug that would reduce mother-child transmission of the HIV virus.[4]

By the late 1980s when Dr. Krisana was appointed director of the research unit at the GPO, HIV infection rates in Thailand had skyrocketed. One oft-cited figure from 1989 reports that 44 percent of Chiang Mai's sex workers were infected with HIV, which spread to their clients—typically heterosexual males—who then spread the disease to their wives, who passed it on to their unborn children, and in such a way caused the disease to proliferate among Thailand's general population.[5] The numbers cited in the play are actually on the low end of the estimates for the 1990s and early 2000s. The pressure on Thailand's government to check the spread of HIV—replicated in *Cocktail*—was particularly acute in the Ministry of Health and the GPO, where Dr. Krisana worked. According to her, most in the GPO thought it impossible that a Thai doctor would find a way to address the pandemic or that it would generate a profit, so they were both incredulous about Dr. Krisana's mission and complacent to continue relying on imported non-generics that most Thais could not afford.

Initially, no other scientist would join Dr. Krisana in her quest because it meant working with poisonous chemicals used to create generic versions of antiretrovirals (ARVs). As a consequence, Dr. Krisana worked alone and even had to test the drugs on herself, causing in one instance an allergic reaction that kept her bedridden for days. Even the play fails to capture those grueling six months of solitary focused exertion, with days beginning at dawn and ending late at night as the persevering Dr. Krisana set out to prove she could create a generic formula for AZT. But those long dark days paid off: she is the person behind the statistics revealing the drastically

---

4. As noted earlier, AZT is a general antiretroviral that is used as a part of normal HIV therapy, not just to treat pregnant women infected with the virus.

5. See for example http://www.avert.org/aidsthai.htm (accessed September 3, 2008).

reduced mother-child transmission figures in Thailand from the mid-1990s on. By 1999, AZT was available at a greatly reduced price and used in most hospitals in Thailand.[6]

As the play reveals, the inexhaustible Dr. Krisana had also to contend with detractors outside the GPO as well. By the late 1990s, hundreds of thousands of individuals in Thailand had contracted the virus, making the need for affordable treatment a national emergency. Dr. Krisana resolved to develop a generic version of the antiretroviral, ddI, which, like AZT, decelerates the speed with which HIV spreads through the body. However, Bristol Myers Squibb, a transnational pharmaceutical giant, had acquired a patent for the tablet form of ddI in the meantime and insisted that Dr. Krisana had broken Thai patent law. They went so far as to pressure their subcontractors to cease supplying Dr. Krisana with the drug. More importantly, Dr. Krisana became indirectly engaged in a lawsuit against BMS that would disclose some of the company's less savory practices. Coincidentally (or not), BMS revoked its patent on ddI and "donated" its patent to Thailand.[7] In the meantime, Dr. Krisana developed the "cocktail" or fixed-dose combination GPO-VIR, a pill that combines three generic ARVs that need only be taken twice a day and was, at the time, eighteen times cheaper than other regimens. The "cocktail" greatly simplified the previously complicated drug regimen for patients who had to take between six and twenty-six pills a day at certain times of the day, sometimes with food, sometimes without, for the rest of their lives. Failure

---

6. Zidovudine, a drug that helps reduce the chances that pregnant mothers would pass on the virus to their children, cost 287 baht per pill in the mid-1990s; Dr. Krisana's generic version was only 8 baht. AZT from the US was 40 baht per pill; Dr. Krisana's was 8 baht. From "Raeron chiwit thi rai chutmai plaithang" (Gypsy Life with No Future), *Sakulthai* 2803 (July 8, 2008), http://www.krisana.org (accessed September 4, 2008).

7. For the complexities of the cases with BMS, see "Raeron chiwit thi rai chutmai plaithang" (Gypsy Life with No Future). See also an excellent article by Tina Rosenberg that offers a global view of the complexities involved in trade patents between transnational pharmaceutical companies and relatively poor countries facing AIDS crises. Tina Rosenberg, "Look at Brazil," *New York Times* (January 28, 2001), www.nytimes.com (accessed September 15, 2007).

to adhere to the schedule could produce more resistant strains of the virus, so Dr. Krisana's three-in-one pill not only eased the treatment regime but also greatly reduced its costs: patients who once paid $474 per month for the non-generic regimen of six pills a day, paid $27 per month for the fixed-dose combination once production of it began in 2002.[8]

Struggle, even if it's successful, can be weary, and certainly Dr. Krisana had had her share of conflict during her years at the GPO. Perhaps these obstacles eased her decision to leave the GPO in 2002 and to commit the rest of her life to Africa. Certainly her work in Thailand had stabilized the AIDS crisis because the GPO produced and distributed cheaper generic drugs. She will tell you that she left because the Thai government promised to help African nations manufacture AIDS drugs, but failed to implement it. She has more recently referred to the huge gap in care between high-income or industrialized countries and care in low-income countries as a "holocaust of the poor" and a "global apartheid of poverty and health."[9] According to a UNAIDS report, 67 percent of all people infected with AIDS in 2007 live in Sub-Saharan Africa, and 75 percent of AIDS deaths in 2007 occurred there.[10] Developing countries such as those in Africa are less able to afford the drugs that treat the disease or the infrastructure and technological expertise to produce the drugs domestically. So when Dr. Krisana received a phone call in 2002 from the owners of a company named Pharmakina operating in the Democratic Republic of Congo (DRC) asking her to help them provide medicines for their employees suffering from HIV/AIDS and malaria, Dr. Krisana agreed immediately.

---

8. Dr. Krisana Kraisintu, "Local Resources for Global Remedies: Increasing Access Towards a Sustainable HIV/AIDS Solution," Asian Social Issues Program, March 3, 2005, New York City, http://www.asiasource.org/asip/kraisintu.cfm (accessed March 14, 2007).
9. Krisana, "Local Resources for Global Remedies."
10. UNAIDS, "2008 Report on the Global AIDS Epidemic," http://data.unaids.org/pub/GlobalReport/2008/jc1510_2008_global_report_pp29_62_en.pdf (accessed October 2, 2008).

One important fact at the time eluded Dr. Krisana: Bukavu, the city in which Pharmakina operates, was at the heart of a conflict zone. Dr. Krisana stepped into a war that had been raging, off and on, since the DRC (named Zaire from 1960 until 1997) gained independence in 1960.[11] Bukavu is the capital of Kivu, a region in the eastern Congo that borders the tiny countries of Rwanda and Burundi. By 1964, the eastern Congo, where Dr. Krisana would eventually reside, broke out in rebellion that ended with over one million deaths and with the beginning of over thirty years of corrupt dictatorship under Joseph Mobutu. Because of the autonomy exercised in Kivu and the instability of Zaire's central government, the country was susceptible to involvement in neighboring wars including the Rwandan civil war. The extent of involvement by neighboring groups, themselves divided into factions, and the number of factions from within the DRC involved in this conflict is bewildering. Angola, Zimbabwe, Chad, and Namibia, in addition to Rwanda, Burundi, and Uganda, were all involved in the Congo imbroglio, where each turned the DRC into zones of control for the extraction of minerals and other natural resources. Kivu has continued to be wracked by violence, rival militias, proxy forces, local warlordism, and plundering.

Dr. Krisana arrived in 2002, one year after the assassination of the DRC's President Kabila and replacement by his son. The war raged on in the jungles surrounding the pharmaceutical factory she designed for Pharmakina, a company purchased by a German named Horst Gebbers and a Frenchman named Etienne Erny in 1999 as conflict again erupted in Kivu. Instead of shutting down the company during the interminable war as the vast majority of other major companies in the area had done, Gebbers and Erny kept their doors open, which meant that they continued to employ hundreds of local staff, who in turn kept their families relatively well fed by comparison to their less fortunate neighbors. Pharmakina owned cinchona plantations:

---

11. This summary of the DRC's combustible history is taken from Martin Meredith, *The Fate of Africa: A History of Fifty Years of Independence* (NY: Public Affairs, 2005), chapters 6, 17, and 28. This is, incidentally, Dr. Krisana's favorite political history of Africa.

the microclimate in Kivu makes it a perfect place to grow chinchona trees, the bark of which is harvested for quinine, an anti-malaria agent. During the war, Pharmakina cornered over one third of the world market for quinine salts.[12] The bold move to keep operations open during the height of the conflict, mass killing, mass rape, and other crimes perpetrated against Kivu's local population indicates something about those who run Pharmakina, which was not exempt from the violence.[13] Theirs is a model of community engagement and commitment, motivated not just by profit but by humane goals. They felt early on that Pharmakina needed to provide medicines for their employees, many of whom suffered not just from malaria but also from AIDS. Dr. Krisana was key to their ability to develop generic antiretrovirals that are now used to treat not just Pharmakina employees, but are made available to the entire DRC population.

From this stepping stone in the DRC, Dr. Krisana launched her life mission in other countries in Africa, which by 2008 included Benin, Burkina Faso, Burundi, Ethiopia, Eritrea, The Gambia, Kenya, Liberia, Mali, Senegal, Tanzania, Uganda, and Zambia. She has inexhaustible energy when it comes to her work in Africa, where facing major drug company resistance, as she did in Thailand, is a comparatively minor obstacle. In Liberia, the poorest country in which she works, the GDP per capita is $400 a year, placing all drugs financially out of reach of the majority of the population. Even so the risk of diseases like malaria, HIV/AIDS, and other illnesses including diarrhea ensures that the median life expectancy there is forty-one years. In 2008, Dr. Krisana trained Liberians how to make anti-malarials. Her work

---

12. Bastian Birkenhäger, "A Beacon of Stability in a Sea of Unrest: The Case of PHARMAKINA in the DRC," written for the UN Global Compact Learning Forum, www.unglobalcompact.org/NewsandEvents/event_archives/ghana_2006/Pharmakina.pdf (accessed August 25, 2008).
13. In 1996, prior to the takeover by Gebbers and Erny, one of many militant groups operating in the area attacked the company, destroying equipment and interrupting the supply of raw materials from the plantations, some of which are located far from the company center. See Birkenhäger.

has also been successful in Tanzania where AIDS-related deaths were estimated to reduce the life expectancy there from sixty-five to thirty-seven years by 2010,[14] and where approximately 140,000 children are living with AIDS.[15] By transferring the technology and formulas for generic antiretrovirals and anti-malarials to Tanzania Pharmaceutical Industries, Dr. Krisana helped the company manufacture these drugs at affordable local prices. These are examples from just two of the African nations with which she works.

It is no wonder then that Vince LiCata and Ping Chong jumped at the chance to write and produce a play about Dr. Krisana's life.[16] For Chong, Dr. Krisana's life experience is the classic David and Goliath story in which a single person, against all odds, personally changes the world. Ping Chong and Vince LiCata met in the early 1990s at the University of Minnesota when LiCata, a post-doc in molecular biology, successfully auditioned for a part in the play, "Persuasion," an adaptation of the controversial young-adult book, *The Chocolate War*, directed by artist-in-residence Chong. For LiCata, Chong was a natural choice as director and cowriter for his vision of a new play that would bring the drama of science to the stage.

A graduate of Johns Hopkins and now professor of biochemistry at Louisiana State University–Baton Rouge, Professor LiCata has two long-term interests that seem, in retrospect, to have ensured that his path would cross that of Dr. Krisana. LiCata researches a family of proteins called Pol I polymerase in which HIV reverse transcriptase, the protein with which Dr. Krisana works, is a family member. In addition, LiCata manifests a happy marriage of science and art in the plays and essays he writes about compelling and humanistic stories behind some of science's greatest achievements. For

---

14. Krisana, "Local Resources for Global Remedies."

15. UNAIDS, "2008 Report on the Global AIDS Epidemic: United Republic of Tanzania, Epidemiological Factsheet Update on HIV and AIDS," http://www.who.int/globalatlas/ predefinedReports/EFS2008/full/EFS2008_TZ.pdf (accessed October 2, 2008).

16. The following section is developed from phone interviews with Mr. Ping Chong and Professor Vince LiCata on August 27, 2008, and August 20, 2008, respectively.

him, writing plays—which he has done since 1990—exercises an entirely different part of his brain than that engaged by biochemistry.

When he contacted Chong about the idea of producing a play based on science, he presented several options, most of which revolved around the little-known but potentially revolutionary achievements of women in science. One focused on Madame Marie-Anne Lavoisier, wife of the "Father of Modern Chemistry" Antoine Lavoisier, who is best known for discovering the role of oxygen in combustion. She is suspected of exerting a strong intellectual force behind her husband's scientific achievements. LiCata also pitched to Chong the controversial story (and subject of LiCata's most recent play) of the discovery of the double helix structure of DNA, credited to James Watson and Francis Crick, but based on the data produced by Rosalind Franklin, who was not recognized for her contributions during her lifetime.

Dr. Krisana is in good scientific company, but her story—more than that of Lavoisier and Franklin—captivated director Chong, whose record of producing socially engaged theater is well known. Chong is a third-generation theater person who grew up in Chinatown in New York City, graduated from the School of Visual Arts and the Pratt Institute, and cut his teeth as a theater performing artist in NY during the radical 1960s. Since then, he has produced over fifty works for the stage, many of which explore the impact of history, culture, and race on the lives of individuals. The life of Dr. Krisana, a Thai woman working in Africa to provide affordable medicines for the poor and committed to teaching Africans how to produce their own generic drugs, intensely and immediately appealed to him. The plays he directs have a message and this one cannot help but inspire viewers: one person can make a difference. Dr. Krisana single-handedly has saved millions of lives, personally changing mortality rates not just in Africa, but in Thailand as well. Dr. Krisana's story grabbed him because she, like him, has devoted her life to the pursuit of social justice. However, for Chong, Dr. Krisana's personal qualities also offered something extremely rare. She is, in short, not just a female hero, not just an Asian female hero, but rather an "Asian alpha female hero." Dr. Krisana offered him an opportunity to shatter all of the stereotypical representations of Asian women: docile, fragile, silent, and exotic, adjectives that one would never use to describe Krisana Kraisintu.

Whereas LiCata originally created a fictionalized script about Dr. Krisana's life, Chong insisted that they stick as closely to her real life as possible. When Dr. Krisana flew to New York City to give a talk at The Asia Society in March 2005, Chong and LiCata met with her. The marathon twelve-hour interview and follow-up emails were fed through LiCata's ingenious brain, which generated a version of the script that Chong and he passed back and forth until it was complete. The perfect *Cocktail* was the result.

Chong and LiCata collaborated synergistically, bringing together very different but highly complementary abilities to *Cocktail*, which was funded by the National Endowment for the Arts, Louisiana State University, the Baton Rouge Performing Arts Center, and the Sloan Foundation. LiCata is the source of the science in the play—the formulas that flash by on the screen in the background, the scenes involving pill pressing and crushing, the accessible descriptions of antiretrovirals. In contrast, Chong's visual arts, dance, and film background bring a highly unusual set of elements to *Cocktail*, including a sound track (something he pioneered for use in plays), multimedia projections such as digital animation, and flawlessly choreographed scenes involving every body, ambulatory or not, on stage. But theirs is not strict division between the artist and the scientist, as demonstrated by LiCata's playwriting skills and tongue-in-cheek article "When Britney Spears Comes to My Lab"[17] and by Chong's technical proficiency as a movement, lighting, and sound expert. Together they have created a mesmerizing experience of Dr. Krisana's life.

To avoid the uni-dimensionality of reading as opposed to watching a live version of the play, readers of *Cocktail* must use their imagination.[18] For

---

17. Vince LiCata, "When Britney Spears Comes to My Lab," *Nature* 451/3 (January 2008), 106.

18. There is an interview with Ping Chong on YouTube that contains clips from the play. See http://www.youtube.com/watch?v=zHq6TN2xkHs (accessed August 28, 2008).

example, the play uses "intelligent lights" which are lights programmed to move on stage as if they too are part of the cast. Green spots highlight the AIDS patients, vibrating frenetically on their bodies, which move in synchronized motion about the stage. In one riveting scene, gurneys, doctors, patients, and the disease itself swing, swerve, and shudder while doctors announce robotically "It is 1990. You are AIDS case number 114,324," and a ticking time bomb crescendos in the background as the years progress and numbers skyrocket. Pressure-cooker intensity created out of organized chaos offers one of Chong's signature scenes of sound and motion, made conceptually meaningful with the scientific substance provided by LiCata. It also captures the mood in Thailand among those, like Dr. Krisana, who understood the dire need to intervene in the AIDS crisis rocking Thailand. The scene shocks the viewer with the reality that the AIDS epidemic in Thailand in the 1990s required Dr. Krisana's heartfelt commitment and practical pharmaceutical know-how to help contain the pandemic. *Cocktail* is an inspiring story of one woman's determination to confront seemingly insurmountable obstacles. In the process of overcoming them, she proves them surmountable after all.

Artists' Statement

Why should I care to know about this person's life?
Because this person made a profound difference in the lives of others.

What is real in *Cocktail*? All the events, all the science, all of the people. What is not real in *Cocktail*? Most of the dialogue is invented, although it is peppered with real quotes from real people. The timeline has been altered in a few places due to theatrical constraints. A few names have been changed to protect the infamous.

Our vision for *Cocktail* is truly a shared vision, a collaborative stretch for both of us. Vince suggested the project because of his interest in portraying real science on stage. Ping was immediately attracted to the project because of its exploration of social justice and its connection to both Asian and African culture. We both have become enraptured, enamored, in-awe-of Krisana Kraisintu. At the start of this project, we spent two days with Krisana. It was a lesson in humility. She has boundless energy, and a depth and drive to her commitment to bring HIV-therapy to the world that is almost super-human in its purity and intensity. We have all read about historical super-human figures: Albert Schweitzer, Mother Teresa, Martin Luther King. But there are less well known superheroes working among us right now: Paul Farmer in Haiti, Eloan dos Santos Pinheiro in Brazil, all the doctors of Médecins sans Frontières, and Krisana. Their names are less recognizable, but they are no less super-human. To spend two days interviewing such an amazing person, to see her near single-minded drive, her searing intelligence, her amazing open-heartedness, is a truly life-changing experience. A large part of why we have created this play is to share Krisana with a wider audience, and to honor her selflessness.

We want to accomplish a variety of goals with this play. We want to create a new type of collaborative theater piece, and we both want to grow intellectually and artistically as a result of creating *Cocktail*. We want to create a stage work that integrates science with stylized staging and movement, and that addresses some very serious global issues. *Cocktail* is a kinetic, lyrical, mystical, but honest and accurate exploration of how one woman invented a new pharmaceutical product under conditions that were anything but conducive: in a recalcitrant government lab and the jungles of Africa in the midst of civil war.

As far as we know, this is the first professionally produced play cowritten by a professional artist and a professional scientist. Some of our early meetings on this project were concerned with how to explain a carbon-carbon bond, or what the difference is between a molecule and an atom. We found a common ground for communication in strange and sometimes crude analogies. A chair is like a molecule: the individual pieces of wood are the individual atoms while the nails or the glue holding the wood pieces together represent the chemical bonds. This is not a great analogy, but it was the one that worked for us in that early session. An analogy that actually made its way into the play is the comparison between HIV reverse transcriptase (HIV-RT) and a Xerox machine.

Upon observing the working routine in Vince's lab, Ping compared the hands-on manipulations performed in the laboratory to a Japanese tea ceremony: the precision of movement, the exact placement of the laboratory vessels and the instruments for transferring and mixing the chemical solutions. It is this type of cross-talk that we are learning to speak. This fusion between art and science is what we want to ultimately present on stage.

Thus, our intent for *Cocktail* is multifold. We want to raise public awareness of the work of Krisana Kraisintu. We want to communicate accurate details about HIV drug manufacture and development. We want to create an awareness of the HIV treatment problems faced by the developing world. We want to give audiences a story and a performance that they find emotionally and intellectually compelling, and create an accessible and memorable play. Above all, the intent of *Cocktail* is to remind all of us that every single one of us has the capacity to make the world a better and more humane place to live.

COCKTAIL

by

Vince LiCata and Ping Chong

Cocktail premiered on April 20, 2007 at Louisiana State University's Swine Palace Theatre, with Michael Tick serving as Producing Artistic Director, and Kristin Sosnowsky, as Managing Director in Baton Rouge, LA. The production was produced in association with Ping Chong & Company and Bruce Allardice, Managing Director in New York, with the support of the National Endowment for the Arts.

CAST

Mia Katigbak	Krisana Kraisintu
Caleb Sekeres	Dr. Bhunbhu, MP Patiset, and Horst Gebbers
Other parts	LSU Ensemble

Director	Ping Chong
Scenic Designer	James L. Murphy
Lighting Designer	Darren McCroom
Sound Designer	EunJin Cho
Costume Designer	Polly Boersig
Projection Designer	Jan Hartley
Production Stage Manager	Karli Henderson

SCENES

CHARACTERS

(IN ORDER OF APPEARANCE)

A minimum of nine actors is necessary, as this is the largest number on stage simultaneously. However, a cast size of twelve to fourteen will allow for faster transitions between busy scenes.

Grandmother
Young Krisana
Farmer
Decha
Prostitute
New Orleans people (5 to 7)
Selena Scott (4; played by a
    distinctly different actress in
    each appearance)
Doctors (8; the same actor can
    play multiple doctors, or a
    doctor and a patient)
Patients (7)
Dr. Krisana
Dr. Bhunbhu
Tido
MPs 1 and 2
Achara
Parents 1 and 2 (mother and
    father)
Nui
Girl
Mother
Panda

Chorus (up to 6)
MP Patiset
Restaurant wait staff (up to 3)
Restaurant customers (2)
Mr. Smythe
Staff 1 (Kitiphan)
Staff 2 (Chuchit)
Staff 3 (Thatsani)
Staff 4, 5, and 6
Director Likhit
Date People 1 and 2
Brighton Miles Pharmaceuticals
    executives (BMP) (6)
Session Chair
Conferees (4 speaking, others as
    possible)
Health Minister's staff (2)
Health Minister
Horst Gebbers
Dirk Gebbers
Extras at airport (up to 5)
Mango
Soldiers (5)
Yosef

SETS AND PROPS

Sets should be as simple and minimal as possible. In the premiere production the floor of the set was white acrylic with volumetric markings (like a lab beaker) along one edge. The upstage wall was completely covered by a projection screen, a trapezoidal shape with the larger dimension at the top.

Rolling tables and stools were used for all furniture pieces in all on-stage scenes (a total of five tables and seven stools was easily manageable). For shadow-play scenes, a platform was constructed behind the projection screen. Furniture used in the shadow plays included a table, a desk, two chairs, and a rocking chair. Upon Dr. Krisana's arrival in Africa (scene 19), approximately twenty potted palm trees (made of newspaper) were brought onstage and remained in place.

There should be minimal or no blackouts/transitions between scenes—the action should be as continuous as possible.

For the laboratory bench in scene 10, Making the Pill, one of the rolling tables was used and was covered with lab equipment and chemical bottles obtained on loan from the local university. The pill press used in the premiere production was a single tablet manual press, also a loan from the local university, although the manufacturer (GlobePharma) also offered a low-cost lease. The press used in the premiere production can be viewed at: http://www.globepharma.com/html/manual_tab__machine.html. This scene can be staged with any available pill press. A manual, portable pill press, also used in the Africa scenes, is available from www.vitapress.com. This small hand press can be used for both scenes if a larger press is not available for scene 10.

Other props, where necessary, were minimal and stylized (e.g., oversized menus in the restaurant). The molecular model in scene 12, High Noon, was constructed from a standard organic chemistry molecular modeling set.

Projected images and movies used in the premiere production are available from the authors (see copyright page for contact information).

PRESET

Sound: Water droplets, one every two to three seconds.

Projection: Preset title "COCKTAIL" on screen, changing colors slowly. House lights fade out. Title fades out.

SCENE 1. ON SAMUI I (SHADOW PLAY)

Sound: Fade in ocean roar.

Projection: Fade in of pan across a map of Pacific Ocean to Thailand, zoom in on Samui Island.

Sound: Quiet Thai music fades in under ocean, then the ocean fades out leaving only the music to play by itself.

Projection: Text "THAILAND, The Island of Samui, 1957" (in English and Thai over the map. Fade out map and leave text up).

Shadow play and digital scenery except for the table and chair. Clouds passing. A Buddhist nun is sitting under a banana palm by a bamboo table fanning herself with a palm fan in shadow play.

As the lights come up on the shadow play, Grandmother is chanting the Buddhabhivadana (the chant for Preliminary Reverence for the Buddha in Theravada Buddhism). Approximate phonetic transliteration: "Namo thassa Bhagavato Arahato Samma Sambuddhassa." *She repeats it three times.*

YOUNG KRISANA. *(She is five years old.)* Grandmother! Grandmother!
Grandmother turns and looks off.
GRANDMOTHER. I'm here, Krisana.

Krisana appears as a child.
YOUNG KRISANA. What are you doing, Grandmother?
GRANDMOTHER. (*Amused*) Why, as you can see I'm resting, my child.
YOUNG KRISANA. Can I rest with you, too?
GRANDMOTHER. You can be with me whenever you like.
Krisana joins her grandmother, but is soon distracted by an insect.

Sound: Music cross-fades with ambient sounds of the tropics, birds, insects. A farmer approaches, on foot, with a basket of produce. Krisana squats beside Grandmother. Seconds pass. Krisana and Grandmother turn toward the sound of the farmer approaching.

FARMER. Sawatdi khrap (*folds hands and bows*).
Grandmother folds hands to receive his bow.
YOUNG KRISANA. Sawatdi kha.
GRANDMOTHER. What do you have today?
FARMER. Potatoes, water spinach, onions, cabbage, squash. The squash are very tasty this time of year. What would you like?
GRANDMOTHER. I will take everything.
FARMER. Everything! You want everything?
GRANDMOTHER. Yes, everything. You can put them on this table. (*Farmer starts putting the vegetables on the table.*) Krisana, help him put the vegetables on the table.
FARMER. (*To himself*) Everything. She wants everything.
GRANDMOTHER. Is this enough? (*She gives money to Krisana, and Krisana gives it to the farmer.*)
FARMER. Oh, yes, Madame, more than enough. Let me give you change.
Grandmother waves to indicate "no change."
FARMER. (*Folds hands and bows*) Khopkhun khrap, Khopkhun khrap. Have a good day.
They watch the farmer leave. Krisana picks up some of the vegetables and plays with them.

7

YOUNG KRISANA. Grandmother?

GRANDMOTHER. Yes, Krisana?

YOUNG KRISANA. Are you very hungry today?

GRANDMOTHER. Am I hungry? Why do you ask?

YOUNG KRISANA. Why did you buy all the farmer's vegetables? Are you going to eat them all by yourself?

GRANDMOTHER. (*Chuckles*) Oh no, Krisana. No. I bought all the farmer's vegetables so he wouldn't have to go all the way to the market, because farmers work very, very hard. I bought these vegetables not only for myself, but for the poor people in our village who can't afford to buy them. Krisana—

YOUNG KRISANA. Yes, Grandmother.

GRANDMOTHER. Listen to me. You must remember that there are people in this world less fortunate than you. So we must help them from time to time. This is what the Buddha teaches us, to be kind to all living things. That is why I devoted my life to the Buddha. (*Sound: Bourbon Street jazz fades in as Grandmother is talking. Jungle sounds fade out.*) If you have enough in your life then you must share with those who have less than you. Never forget that, Krisana.

YOUNG KRISANA. Yes, Grandmother.

GRANDMOTHER. Never forget . . . (*echoes into silence*).

Fade to black.

SCENE 2. PATIENT ZERO

Sound: Bourbon Street jazz gets louder. Sound of trolley or occasional car going by.

Projection: Text "NEW ORLEANS, 1981" with image of Bourbon Street.

Decha enters. Prostitute enters. Three people cross, laughing. Decha and the prostitute watch the people in the street. A couple in love walk by. A drunkard attempts to pick up a cigarette. The prostitute approaches Decha.

PROSTITUTE. Got the time?

DECHA. It's almost midnight.

PROSTITUTE. Where you from, honey?

DECHA. Thailand—Bangkok.

PROSTITUTE. Bangkok. Wow. You know I've always loved that name, Bangkok.

DECHA. Excuse me?

PROSTITUTE. You know, Bang—Cock? Get it?

DECHA. In Thai it means "City of the Angels."

PROSTITUTE. What you doing all the way over here, honey? (*unwraps gum*)

DECHA. I'm starting grad school in a week.

PROSTITUTE. No shit? Ain't that something. (*Pause*) You seem kind of lonely. (*Pause, no answer. Tosses the gum wrapper*) You know, I got a sure-fire cure for the blues, honey, and it'll only set you back $50.

DECHA. $50?

PROSTITUTE. Yeah, $50. How about it, honey?

DECHA. (*Considers*) Okay.

PROSTITUTE. What's your name? Mine is Desiree.

DECHA. I am Decha.

PROSTITUTE. Decha?

DECHA. Yes, Decha.
PROSTITUTE. Nice name.
    They exit.

Fade to black.

Sound: Bourbon Street jazz fades out.

SCENE 3. BBC 1

*Sound and projection: TV channel switches. Clips from Thai TV shows flip past,
eventually stopping at the BBC newscast. News story icon in upper cor-
ner of newscast screen shows the words, "Thai Patient Zero?" with a
BBC logo. (The character of Selena Scott should be played by a different actress in each of the BBC newscasts in the play.)*

SELENA SCOTT. Good evening. I'm Selena Scott and this is the BBC
World Service for October 22, 1984. The Ramathibodi Hospital
in Bangkok today reported the first confirmed case of AIDS in
Thailand: a thirty-year-old Thai graduate student who, according
to the report, contracted the infection in New Orleans, Louisiana,
approximately three years previously. He is reported to be in
poor condition. In related news, researchers in the United States
announced that they have begun development of a commercial
test for the virus believed to be responsible for AIDS. Currently,
the Center for Disease Control in Atlanta, Georgia, remains one
of the only reliable AIDS diagnostic facilities worldwide. In other
news—*(screen and sound go to static)*

Sound: Static bumps out. Ticking starts.

SCENE 4. PATIENTS & DOCTORS

Sound: Whispers and music fade in. Ticking continues.

Projection: A giant HIV virus slowly begins rising, like a sun, throughout the scene.

> *Throughout the scene patients are brought on and off using tables with wheels that function as beds. Sometimes there are multiple beds on stage, sometimes only one. Decha is sitting up on one of the tables as if it were a hospital bed, looking at his arms. A doctor enters. All doctors wear dark blue scrubs or lab coats. All patients wear light green patient gowns. Green dots are projected onto all of the patients, and late in the scene, onto one of the doctors.*

DECHA. What's wrong with me, Doctor? What is this? What are these spots on my arms? *(repeats it twice, continuing to look at spots on his arms)*
Projection: Green dots of light play across Decha's body.

DOCTOR 1. You have AIDS. You have a virus. You have a communicable disease. Stay right where you are, young man. Do not move. (*He shouts.*) Nurse. Nurse! I need to know everyone who has been in contact with this patient. Nurse! Nurse!

DECHA. What's wrong with me, Doctor? What is this? What are these spots?

Sound: Loud buzzer.

> *Decha continues to ask the doctor about spots even as his bed is pushed offstage. Another table with wheels is brought on in a choreographic manner.*

PATIENT 2. What is it, Doctor? What do I have?

DOCTOR 2. You have tested positive for AIDS.

PATIENT 2. What is AIDS?

DOCTOR 2. It is a dangerous virus. It is a communicable disease.

PATIENT 2. Can you stop it? Can you help me?

DOCTOR 2. Nothing can be done. We have no treatment for this yet.

DOCTOR 3. There is some talk about a new drug being developed in the United States, something called AZT.

Projection: The chemical structure of AZT appears on screen, along with the text "AZT". The image fades out almost immediately.

DOCTOR 3. (*Continues*) But, we do not have this drug here in Thailand.

PATIENT 2. Doctor, what's going to happen to me?

DOCTOR 2. You are going to die. (*Pause*) This is 1985, and you are Thai AIDS case number 408.

Sound: Loud buzzer, music bumps out under the Dr. Bhunbhu and Dr. Krisana segments.

We see Dr. Bhunbhu at a desk in an office.

DR. BHUNBHU. Dr. Kraisintu, thank you for responding so promptly.

DR. KRISANA. Please, call me Krisana.

Secretary brings them tea, and immediately exits.

DR. BHUNBHU. Have you considered my offer on behalf of the Thai government?

DR. KRISANA. I have, but I . . .

DR. BHUNBHU. Good, good. As you know, there are only a handful of pharmaceutical chemists in Thailand at this time. You are one of the few, and perhaps the most qualified. You have done excellent work here. That is why I am so excited you are interested in this new position. Have you given our proposal much thought, Dr. Kraisintu?

Sound: Loud buzzer, music bumps in and ticking bumps out.

PATIENT 3. What are you trying to tell me? Doctor? Doctor. (*Pause; the doctor ignores him/her, writing something on the patient's chart.*)

TIDO. (*Off to the side of the stage, he is talking on a phone. He says the first line in German, repeats it in English, then continues in English*): Ja, ja, die Situation ist schrecklich hier! Yes, yes, the situation is terrible here. Pretty much what I expected. Yes, I'm at the hospital now. I came here directly. Let me say goodnight to Elke.

PATIENT 3. What are you trying to tell me? Doctor? What do you mean?

TIDO. Elke? Hello, sweetheart! I'm in Thailand . . . Yes . . . I'm in a place called Thailand. Yes. Thailand. No, it's very different from Germany.

PATIENT 3. What are you trying to tell me? That there is no hope? Is that what you are trying to tell me?

TIDO. Daddy misses you too, sweetheart. More than you know. But there are people here who need my help.

PATIENT 3. I don't understand.

TIDO. Yes, sweetheart, I know you need me, too.

PATIENT 3. I don't understand. Are you telling me that there is no hope?

DOCTOR 3. That is correct.

DOCTOR 4. This is 1986, and you are Thai AIDS case number 2,201.

TIDO. (*Singing Brahms lullaby in German into the phone*)
    Guten Abend, gute Nacht, Von Englien bewacht
    Die zeigen im Traum, dir Christkindleins Baum
    Schlaf nun selig und sues, Schau im Traum's Paradies
    Schlaf nun selig und sues, Schau im Traum's Paradies

PATIENT 3. Doctor? Can I tell you something? Doctor?
    Patient 3 is wheeled offstage.

Sound: Loud buzzer, music out, ticking.

DR. KRISANA. Dr. Bhunbhu, I am honored by your offer, but I am worried that—

DR. BHUNBHU. Dr. Kraisintu, your work here at the GPO for the past several years has been exemplary. Exemplary! But now we want the Thai Government Pharmaceutical Organization to earn its name—as you know, we currently make very few pharmaceuticals at all. All these skin creams, shampoos, and toothpastes—well, we had to start somewhere. But now it is time to move forward. Have you given our proposal much thought, Dr. Kraisintu?

DR. KRISANA. Please, call me Krisana.

Sound: Loud buzzer, music in, ticking out.

PATIENT 4. Tell my parents anything but don't tell them I have AIDS. Please don't tell them I have AIDS. Please. Don't tell them I have . . . (*Repeats twice, overlapping the following dialogue*).

DOCTOR 5. There is a new drug called AZT.

Projection: The chemical AZT appears on screen again, then fades out.

DOCTOR 5. (*Continues*) But it is very expensive. Not even I could afford it.

DOCTOR 3. This is 1987, and you are Thai AIDS case number 22,898.

PATIENT 4. Don't tell them. Please don't tell them. (*Repeat, fades to a whisper*).

Two MPs enter. Patient 5 is wheeled in, and is crying quietly.

MP 1. (*The two MPs speak to each other*). The government does not believe that Thais can give AIDS to other Thais. The government believes that only Westerners can infect other Thais. Why? Because this is an imported disease.

MP 2. Of course, that's it! How stupid of me.

TIDO. (*Speaking to Doctor 5*) Mein Gott. This is 1988. Ignorance and indifference have allowed this disease to take hold of your country.

Listen to these two (*indicates the MPs*). And they're Members of Parliament! We now know AIDS is caused by the HIV virus. We are now learning to treat HIV.

DOCTOR 5. (*To Tido*) I know that, and you know that, but there is no money for research or treatment. Our government spent less than $200,000 this year on AIDS. Government spending on AIDS in the United States this year was more than 1 billion dollars. Our government has to do more, but they don't want to do more. (*To the patient*) I will do what I can to help you.

MP 1. (*Speaking to MP 2*) There is a simple solution to all of this. We'll just have to keep Western tourists out of Thailand. It's clear they are the problem.

MP 2. My thoughts exactly!

MP 1. It's that simple. We have to be going—the parliamentary session starts in an hour. (*Starts to walk away*)

MP 2. (*To MP 1*) Wait a minute, wait a minute, if the tourists are kept out of Thailand, then the sex industry will collapse! That's a lot of money!

MPs 1 AND 2. (*Simultaneously*) I think we have a problem.

DOCTOR 5. (*To the patient*) I think we have a very serious problem. This is 1988 and you are Thai AIDS case number 62,107.

Sound: Loud buzzer, music out, ticking in.

DR. BHUNBHU. We are offering you the position of Director of Research and Development. This is a new position within the GPO.

DR. KRISANA. This is a tremendous honor, but I . . .

DR. BHUNBHU. You will have your own laboratories, you will have your own personnel, and you will have 250 million baht for new equipment exclusively for your work. And you can recruit staff of your own choosing.

DR. KRISANA. I'd like to . . .

DR. BHUNBHU. Do you accept the position? On behalf of the Thai people, what do you say, Dr. Kraisintu?

DR. KRISANA. I've given your offer a great deal of thought, Dr. Bhunbhu.

DR. BHUNBHU. *(On the edge of his seat)* And, Dr. Kraisintu?

DR. KRISANA. I will accept your offer . . .

DR. BHUNBHU. Excellent!

DR. KRISANA. . . . on one condition.

Sound: Loud buzzer, music in, ticking out.

Patient 6 appears lifeless on his bed.

PARENT 1 (MOTHER). Son, can you hear me? . . . Mother's here. Your sister, Nui, is here, too. See? Son?

DOCTOR 6. I'm sorry. I don't think he can hear you.

PARENT 1. *(To Nui)* Talk to him, Nui. You know how much he misses you.

NUI. Somchai, we want you to get well soon. You can do it. I know you can do it.

PARENT 2 (FATHER). *(To Tido)* Why does it say "Tuberculosis Ward" outside my son's room?

TIDO. Because the Thai government does not want to admit that AIDS is a national problem.

PARENT 2. Who are you?

TIDO. I am from Doctors Without Borders. We're just trying to help.

DOCTOR 5. *(Enters)* Dr. Tido! I could use your help—there's a case we want you to look at.

TIDO. Certainly, certainly. *(They both exit.)*

DOCTOR 6. *(To Nui)* I don't think he can hear you anymore.

NUI. Somchai, you can't leave us so soon.

PARENT 1. Son, wake up. Son, wake up.

DOCTOR 6. Visiting hours are over.

PARENT 1. *(Screams)* Wake up! Son, Wake up!

DOCTOR 6. This is 1990, and you are Thai AIDS case number 114,324.

Sound: Several glasses crash on the floor and shatter. Music continues.

PARENT 1. Wake up, Somchai. Please wake up. Please. Please (*continues, slowly trailing off as she is led offstage by her husband*).

PATIENT 7. (*Appears lifeless, then sits up suddenly*) I'm feeling much better. My sight came back. I don't have the diarrhea anymore. My hearing came back. I actually took a walk in the corridor today without a walker. I think in a few weeks I'm going to be just fine. Doctor?

DOCTOR 7. (*Looks up from clipboard*) Yes?

PATIENT 7. I, ah . . . just . . . I was, I, um, what if, um . . . will my wife become infected, too?

DOCTOR 7. You should have thought about that before you fucked that prostitute. You are Thai AIDS case number 228,654.

DOCTOR 8. (*To Doctor 7 as other doctors all begin to enter*) If the government does not start doing something about HIV and AIDS soon, all of Thailand will become infected. Somehow we have to get people to use condoms. Last year there were 140,000 new cases in Thailand alone. It's a nightmare.

DOCTOR 4. You are Thai AIDS case number 230,988.

DOCTOR 6. You are Thai AIDS case number 248,628.

DOCTOR 5. You are Thai AIDS case number 300,107.

DOCTORS 3, 5. You are Thai AIDS case number 316,394.

DOCTOR 7. You are Thai AIDS case number 323,789.

DOCTORS 3, 4, 5, 6. You are Thai AIDS case number 325,111.

DOCTORS 4, 6, 7. You are Thai AIDS case number 343,291.

ALL. You are Thai AIDS case number 352,731.

DOCTORS 4, 5, 6, 7: You are Thai AIDS case number 359,273.

ALL. You are Thai AIDS case number 365,422.

Sound: Loud buzzer, music out, ticking continues.

DR. KRISANA. I've given your offer a great deal of thought, Dr. Bhunbhu, but if I accept, there is one condition.

DR. BHUNBHU. And what is that condition?!

DR. KRISANA. That I be allowed to work on whatever the Thai people need.

DR. BHUNBHU. (*Long pause as he tries to figure out the "catch"*) On whatever the Thai people need? You have my word.

DR. KRISANA. Then I am honored to accept your gracious offer.

DR. BHUNBHU. That's excellent. Absolutely wonderful. (*He picks up the phone and dials an internal number.*) Achara? Yes, could you come to my office for a moment. (*He hangs up the phone.*) I have someone who I'd like you to meet. You don't know how happy you've made me. I was afraid you'd say "no," and join a private company. So tell me, what will you work on first?

DR. KRISANA. Ibuprofen.

DR. BHUNBHU. Hmm . . . Interesting.

Achara runs on, stops short.

DR. BHUNBHU. Dr. Kraisintu, I'd like you to meet Achara Eksaengsri, your new personal administrative assistant.

DR. KRISANA. Your name is Achara?

ACHARA. Yes.

DR. KRISANA. I'm looking forward to working with you.

ACHARA. (*Flustered*) Dr. Kraisintu, I am honored to be your assistant and to assist you . . . in any way that I might . . . assist you.

Dr. Krisana laughs.

Blackout.

Sound: Ticking bumps out and channel switching bumps in.

Projection: The giant HIV virus bumps out.

SCENE 5. BBC 2

Projection: BBC broadcast with background green-screened to add other elements.

Dr. Krisana enters about midway through Selena's report and watches the broadcast.

SELENA SCOTT. . . . making mother to child transmission of AIDS a growing threat not only in Thailand, but also in the bordering countries of Laos and Cambodia. Dr. Tido von Schoen-Angerer, a physician with Doctors Without Borders in Thailand, cited political indifference as one of the key obstacles to progress. Dr. von Schoen-Angerer spoke with us from Bangkok earlier today.

Projection: Image switches to Tido being interviewed.

TIDO. Yes, thank you, Selena. It is Selena, correct? Selena Scott?
SELENA. Yes.
TIDO. Well, Selena, it seems to me that the Thai government remains reluctant to pursue treatment of HIV, which means that many of our patients will quickly develop full-blown AIDS if something is not done. There are existing options, but—
Dr. Krisana points a remote control at the screen and mutes the sound while Tido continues to talk.
DR. KRISANA. Achara?
ACHARA. Yes?
DR. KRISANA. I need you to get me some information. Please get me contact information for Samchully, Aziz, and Ajinomoto.
ACHARA. (*Writing it*) Samchully, Aziz, and um . . .
DR. KRISANA. Ajinomoto.

ACHARA. Aji Nomoto. Yes, of course, right away. (*She starts to exit.*) Um,
Dr. Kraisintu? These are people in the GPO?

DR. KRISANA. No, Achara, they are chemical companies.
They exit. The image switches to static.

SCENE 6. AJINOMOTO COMMERCIAL

Sound: Channel change, static.

Projection: The television image switches through the channels to an Ajinomoto commercial with a pantomiming red panda. After a few seconds the sound mutes, but the commercial keeps playing. At this point the action on stage (below) begins. The Ajinomoto logo comes on screen after the projected commercial finishes and stays till the end of the scene.

GIRL. Mom? Mom. Mom! I'm hungry.

MOTHER. How about some *pad thai?*

GIRL. *Pad thai?* It's my favorite food!

The Ajinomoto panda bear bursts onstage with a large bottle of Ajinomoto MSG. The panda is accompanied by a chorus of six singers. The mother has her back to the panda and the chorus. Only the girl sees them.

PANDA. *Pad thai?* Are you having *pad thai?* Then you need MSG. Ajinomoto MSG!

GIRL. It's Aji-Panda! Aji-Panda!

PANDA AND CHORUS. (*Singing to the tune of "Yankee Doodle"*)
Ah, the best ingredient!
A-ji-nomoto MSG!
Source of flavor, from the Panda.
A-ji-Panda MSG!

GIRL. (*Clapping her hands and laughing in delight*) Aji-Panda! Aji-Panda!

The mother turns and sees the panda as it is shaking MSG onto the pad thai. The girl is helping the panda shake the giant bottle of MSG.

MOTHER. (*Grabs her head and screams in fright, then calms down and speaks*) What in the world is going on here?

GIRL. Mom! Mom! Aji-Panda! Aji-Panda!

MOTHER. Oh, it's Aji-Panda.

The girl, the mother, the panda, and the chorus sing the song together.

GIRL, PANDA, CHORUS. Ah, the best ingredient!

> Aji-nomoto MSG!
>
> Source of flavor from the Panda,
>
> Aji-Panda MSG!

Chorus exits, waving and saying "bye-bye" in cute happy voices. The mother and daughter each take a bite of the pad thai.

GIRL. Mmm . . . Very tasty today!

MOTHER. Wow! It's delicious.

VOICE-OVER (VO). Ajinomoto. The Source of Tomorrow.

The mother, daughter, and panda stay at their table and eat quietly throughout the next scene.

Projection: The Ajinomoto logo onscreen fades into the text "Ajinomoto. The Source of Tomorrow".

SCENE 7. VEGETARIAN RESTAURANT

Sound: Music for restaurant setting. Music fades out when the scene is set and ambient restaurant sound fades in.

Projection: Text "BANGKOK 1991" with image of Bangkok skyline.

We overhear owner of restaurant (MP Patiset) and a group of men laughing in the restaurant. Several other diners fill up other tables. During the course of this, Dr. Krisana enters and overhears their conversation as she is waiting for lunch.

MP Patiset. No, no, no. Oh, I don't think so. It can't possibly be so!

MP 1. I'm afraid it's true, sir.

MP 2. The man actually put a condom on a banana while standing at his desk in the parliament.

MP Patiset. What an embarrassment he is.

MP 1. Mr. Patiset, sir, your restaurant is 100 percent vegetarian, is it not?

MP Patiset. Yes, of course, you know that. But what has this to do with Senator Mechai Viravaidya and his condoms?

MP 1. Well, are you missing any bananas?

MPs 1 and 2 burst into laughter. MP Patiset does not laugh at anything.

MP 2. I don't think Senator Viravaidya is a vegetarian. (*He prods MP 1 to emphasize the joke. MP 1 laughs weakly. When the MPs realize that MP Patiset is not laughing with them, they start to settle down.*) Well, anyway, I don't think you'll see him dining here at your restaurant.

MP Patiset. I don't really care if he dines here or not as long as he votes the way we want him to.

MP 2. Agreed!

MP 1. That's right. It's a shame, though. He's missing out on some of the best food in Bangkok. You do make the best *pad thai* in all of Thailand!

MP 2. I'll second that! The very best!

MP PATISET. Excellent! Thank you! Thank you! You are too kind, Gentlemen. Well, don't let me keep you from your lunch and feel free to order whatever else you like. I've already taken care of the bill.

Disingenuous murmurs of protest from the MPs.

MP 1. Do you think we could have another bottle of . . .

MP PATISET. Of course, of course. Waiter! Another bottle from the new shipment for our esteemed members of parliament, Mr. Alisa and Mr. Karun. I'll see you both at the policy discussion this afternoon. And I hope Senator Viravaidya isn't going to embarrass us again by distributing condoms at today's meeting, too. I really believe he's losing his mind. See you later, Gentlemen.

MPs 1 AND 2. See you later and thanks again for lunch.

MP PATISET. Don't mention it.

MP Patiset, as he passes tables, greets customers he knows, including the Ajinomoto family left from the commercial in scene 6. He speaks in a friendly way to the mother and daughter.

MP PATISET. How is your food?

GIRL. It's delicious.

MP Patiset sees the bottle of MSG on their table and picks it up.

MP PATISET. That's funny. Our food is supposed to be completely MSG free. Hmm.

As MP Patiset passes Dr. Krisana's table, she stops him.

DR. KRISANA. Excuse me, did I hear correctly that you are Mr. Patiset, from the parliament?

MP PATISET. Yes.

DR. KRISANA. I'm Krisana Kraisintu, Director of Research and Development at the Government Pharmaceutical Organization, the GPO.

MP Patiset. Excellent! I'm honored to have you in my restaurant. May I sit down?

Dr. Krisana. Please. Forgive me for eavesdropping, but you do have the best *pad thai* in Bangkok, not to mention the unmentioned, the best green curry, also.

MP Patiset. Excellent! Well, I am an important public figure. I can't be seen to be serving indifferent Thai cuisine. I have to be careful of my image. You probably don't know this, but the prime minister calls me often for my opinion on matters of state. (*Aside to an entering guest*) Hello, how are you today? (*To Dr. Krisana*) I am one of the very few in parliament he confides in. I have access to his direct line.

Dr. Krisana. Really? I had no idea you were that important.

MP Patiset. Did you know I was recently voted best-dressed politician in *Jewels and Diamond* magazine? There were a number of pictures of me. In color! It's still on the newsstands. (*Aside*) Good to have you here again, Mr. Seniwirat. (*To Dr. Krisana*) I can get you a copy.

Dr. Krisana. Oh. That would be . . . um . . . great.

MP Patiset. I'll get you a dozen. I have two hundred copies.

Dr. Krisana. Really? How do you run the People's Dhamma Party, run the restaurant, and still find time to be in *Jewels and Diamond* magazine?

MP Patiset. (*Chuckles, self-satisfied*) Can I offer you some excellent Bordeaux? It's a new shipment.

Dr. Krisana. Oh, thank you, but no. I don't drink alcohol at lunch. I have to go back to the lab—.

MP Patiset. Waiter! (*Gets waiter's attention*) A bottle from the new shipment. Have you ordered yet? You must try the pureed aubergine. Waiter! The pureed aubergine.

At some point during this conversation, the panda and family finish, pay, and leave. Also, at some point Tido and an associate come into the restaurant to eat.

DR. KRISANA. Mr. Patiset, did I hear correctly that Senator Viravaidya was distributing condoms in the parliament?

MP PATISET. Oh my, you do eavesdrop!

DR. KRISANA. Don't worry, we are in the same political party. I have been a member of the People's Dhamma Party for many years.

MP PATISET. Excellent! Senator Viravaidya is mad, of course. They call him the Condom King of Thailand—it is a disgrace. It's bad enough that he's publicly dumped AIDS prevention onto the government's plate. Now he actually wants us to pay for it.

DR. KRISANA. You think it's a bad idea?

MP PATISET. It is a terrible thing. This AIDS (*pause as he searches for a word*) thing.

DR. KRISANA. It certainly is. Then you do support an AIDS prevention program?

MP PATISET. Not at all! AIDS leaves a dirty stain on all of Thailand. Last week, French TV was here and they cornered me and asked me about the AIDS epidemic in Thailand. The AIDS epidemic! Can you imagine?! They could have asked me about the beautiful new sports complex that I cosponsored, or my Beautify Bangkok Campaign, or the excellent cuisine I serve, but no, they have to bring up AIDS here in my very own restaurant. It just wasn't appropriate. As far as I am concerned, I'll be glad when it's all over.

DR. KRISANA. You will be glad when what's over? I don't understand. Is there a new law coming from parliament?

MP PATISET. Oh no, nothing like that. I simply mean when they all die of AIDS.

DR. KRISANA. Excuse me?

MP PATISET. When they all die of AIDS.

A bell rings and everyone in the restaurant turns to one side.

DR. KRISANA. Mr. Patiset, there's an epidemic in Thailand and no one is doing anything about it.

MP PATISET. Let Nature take its course. Let Nature cleanse our country of the degenerates, the drug users, the so-called sex industry. The bad people. Why should the government have to shoulder the responsibility?

DR. KRISANA. I thought our party protected human rights.

MP PATISET. Absolutely. (*Speaks to some patrons at another table*) Are you enjoying your meal? (*Back to Dr. Krisana*) That's correct, but human rights for good people.

DR. KRISANA. But, but, mothers are contracting AIDS, farmers are contracting AIDS, children are contracting AIDS. What about them?

MP PATISET. (*Getting more impatient*) Dr. Kraisintu, you are an intelligent person. Stop and think for a minute. If people are getting AIDS, it is because they are consorting with bad people. That's why they get AIDS. I'm sure you have more important things to do at the GPO than worry about people who get AIDS. Let them die off naturally. (*He sees someone coming and puts on a smiling face.*) Now, if you will excuse me . . .

WAITER. Excuse me, sir, this is Mr. Smythe, with Lifestyles Industries. You asked me to let you know when he arrived.

MP PATISET. Excellent! Thank you for coming to my restaurant. How was your trip, Mr. Smythe? (*Mr. Smythe makes a grimace of exhaustion.*)

MR. SMYTHE. Bloody awful! Twenty-two hour flight.

MP PATISET. Long, I'm sure. Let me get you some new wine that's just arrived. It's a vintage Bordeaux. It goes very well with Thai food. Waiter!

All sound in the restaurant bumps out, and everyone else leaves the stage.

DR. KRISANA. (*Makes a call on her cell phone and a phone begins to ring*) Achara?

ACHARA. Yes, Dr. Kraisintu?

DR. KRISANA. Do I have any meetings scheduled later today?

ACHARA. No, Dr. Kraisintu. But we are waiting for answers from—

DR. KRISANA. Never mind that now. Achara, I want you to draft a letter of resignation for me.

ACHARA. You are resigning from the GPO?

DR. KRISANA. No, no, no. I'm resigning from membership in the People's Dhamma Party. I don't want to belong to it anymore. There is a fool with a head the size of a pumpkin leading it now.

ACHARA. I'll have it ready for your signature when you return.

A stagehand brings Dr. Krisana a yellow lab coat, and she puts it on.

DR. KRISANA. Good. And Achara, please make an appointment for me with the new director. There's something I want to talk to him about.

ACHARA. Very well, Dr. Krisana. Is that all?

DR. KRISANA. Please let the senior staff know that I will be back soon. And Achara, one more thing. Do you remember the Ajinomoto sales representative who visited us last week?

ACHARA. The one who looked like a giant panda?

DR. KRISANA. Yes, yes, that one. Didn't he say they could also make antiretrovirals?

ACHARA. Antiretrovirals? You mean AIDS drugs?

DR. KRISANA. Yes.

ACHARA. Oh, yes, he did say that. I remember it.

DR. KRISANA. Good, good. Please see if you can contact him again.

ACHARA. Of course. Right away.

SCENE 8. STAFF BUZZ

Sound: Bump in ticking and ambient lab sounds.

Projection: The GPO logo appears. A grid of products produced by the Thai GPO appears progressively through the scene.

> *Suddenly people begin coming from all directions converging on Dr. Krisana, speaking as they enter. The staff wear sky blue lab coats. Dr. Krisana wears yellow.*

STAFF 1 (KITIPHAN). Dr. Krisana, the new aspirin formulation is ready to send to production.

STAFF 2 (CHUCHIT). I think we've finally got the dry syrup multivitamin working.

STAFF 3 (THATSANI). The quinine tablet test results are excellent.

STAFF 4. We need your signature.

STAFF 5. Acetominaphen tablets are not storing well. We may need new packaging.

DR. KRISANA. What is the status of the antihistamine syrup development?

STAFF 6. Antihistamine syrup bioequivalence tests are scheduled for next week.

DR. KRISANA. How many volunteers?

STAFF 6. Sixty—half for generic, half for name brand.

DR. KRISANA. Excellent. Diazepam?

STAFF 1 (KITIPHAN). Diazepam?

STAFF 1, 2, 3, 4, 6. (*As though calling out a name, repeatedly*) Diazepam? Diazepam? Diazepam! Diazepam?

STAFF 5. (*Pulls a piece of paper from folder and waves above his/her head*) Diazepam! Diazepam!

DR. KRISANA. (*Takes the paper*) Ah, excellent!

STAFF 1 (KITIPHAN). We need your signature.

STAFF 2 (CHUCHIT). We've been able to make the multivitamin syrup in five different flavors.

STAFF 3 (THATSANI). We need your signature.

STAFF 4. I have the test results for the anti-diabetic formulations.

DR. KRISANA. There is a new anti-diabetic drug from the U.S. Do we have any information on it?

STAFF 5. We need your signature.

STAFF 6. I need you to look over the release forms for the antihistamine tests.

Achara enters and hands Dr. Krisana some papers. The requests and statements from the staff members begin to overlap as Dr. Krisana concentrates more and more on the papers Achara has brought her.

STAFF 1 (KITIPHAN). We need your signature.

STAFF 5. What should we do about the acetominaphen tablets?

STAFF 6. Should the antihistamine bioequivalence volunteers include both men and women?

STAFF 1 AND 3. We need your signature.

STAFF 5. What should we do next?

STAFF 2 (CHUCHIT). We've got rambutan-flavored vitamin syrup, starfruit-flavored, jackfruit-flavored, dragonfruit-flavored, and mango-flavored.

ALL. Ah, mango.

STAFF 3 (THATSANI). We can ship the quinine tablets by next week if you authorize it.

STAFF 4. We need your signature.

DR. KRISANA. (*Stops their clamor with a raise of her hand*) I have a new project, and I'll need several volunteers to form an initial team.

ALL. (*Individually*) What is it? Tell us. A new project? How exciting!

DR. KRISANA. I want to begin making treatments for HIV.

There is a long silence.

STAFF 1 (KITIPHAN). Antiretrovirals?

DR. KRISANA. Yes.

STAFF 2 (CHUCHIT). Antiretrovirals?

DR. KRISANA. Yes.

STAFF 3 (THATSANI). Did you say antiretrovirals?

DR. KRISANA. Yes.

STAFF 4. Anti-HIV antiretrovirals?

DR. KRISANA. Yes.

STAFF 5 AND 6. (*Simultaneously*) Antiretrovirals?

DR. KRISANA. Yes and yes.

STAFF 1 (KITIPHAN). Aaaaaaaaaaah . . . aren't they toxic?

DR. KRISANA. Yes, I believe they are, so we'll need protective clothing, yes. Good thinking, Kitiphan. Achara, what time is my appointment with the new director?

ACHARA. Dr. Likhit said he would see you at four.

DR. KRISANA. Then, that is when I shall return. (*She exits.*)
Achara faces the staff.

ACHARA. Well?

STAFF 1 (KITIPHAN). Well, um, I . . . I have to get back to check on the aspirin (*exits*).

STAFF 6. Yes, and there is still a lot of organization to do for the antihistamine bioequivalency tests (*exits*).

STAFF 2 (CHUCHIT). Well, the multivitamin syrup isn't going to ship itself (*exits*).

STAFF 3 (THATSANI). Did you know that the only source of raw quinine in the entire world is a small factory in Africa? (*exits*).

STAFF 5. Perhaps if we add a bit of desiccant to the acetominaphen bottles—yes, yes, that might help with the storage problem (*exits*).

STAFF 4. (*To Achara after a short pause*) Uh, um . . . I have to go to the bathroom (*exits*).
Achara exits.

(*Note: The following conversation between Dr. Krisana and Dr. Bhunbhu is optional, and may be cut if desired.*)

Cross-cut to a Thai street where Dr. Krisana and Dr. Bhunbhu are walking and talking. He starts to stumble, and she catches him, preventing him from falling into the street.

Sound: A car horn.

DR. KRISANA. Careful, Dr. Bhunbhu!
DR. BHUNBHU. Antiretrovirals? Did you say antiretrovirals?
DR. KRISANA. Yes.

Projection: A large map of Africa begins to drift slowly onstage from the side. It drifts across the GPO product grid.

DR. BHUNBHU. You said antiretrovirals.
DR. KRISANA. That's right, Dr. Bhunbhu.
DR. BHUNBHU. That will be expensive.
DR. KRISANA. Yes.
DR. BHUNBHU. You know that I am officially retired. I've only been staying on to help advise the new director.
DR. KRISANA. Yes, I know, but I thought that—
DR. BHUNBHU. Dr. Kraisintu, I would like you to know how very proud I am of your accomplishments at the GPO over the past few years.
DR. KRISANA. Thank you, Dr. Bhunbhu. That means a lot to me.
DR. BHUNBHU. I'm afraid, however, that antiretrovirals will be difficult. You must get approval from the new director, Dr. Likhit. You know that I have never restricted your work, but it's out of my hands now.
DR. KRISANA. I understand.
DR. BHUNBHU. I will put in a good word, of course, but I'm afraid that's all I can do.
DR. KRISANA. Yes.
DR. BHUNBHU. Good luck.
DR. KRISANA. Thank you.

DR. BHUNBHU. I remember that MP Patiset—you know the one from the People's Dhamma Party—I remember he runs a very nice vegetarian restaurant in one of the buildings near here. I was thinking of having a little *pad thai*. Have you ever been to his restaurant?

DR. KRISANA. Yes, I used to eat there all the time.

DR. BHUNBHU. You used to eat there?

DR. KRISANA. I'm sorry to say the last time I was there, things seemed a bit rotten.

DR. BHUNBHU. Rotten? Oh dear. Well, perhaps some sushi then. Will you join me?

DR. KRISANA. I'd love to, but I have an appointment with Dr. Likhit this afternoon.

DR. BHUNBHU. You never waste time, do you, Krisana? May I call you Krisana?

DR. KRISANA. Of course . . . um . . .

DR. BHUNBHU. Taharn.

DR. KRISANA. Of course, Taharn, my friend.

DR. BHUNBHU. Good luck to you, Krisana. And so long.

DR. KRISANA. (*Pause*) So long.

DR. BHUNBHU. So long.

SCENE 9. DIRECTOR LIKHIT / DR. KRISANA DECIDES TO GO IT ALONE

Sound: Cross bump from traffic to ticking.

Projection: Africa is still drifting across the GPO product grid.

DIRECTOR LIKHIT. Profits, Dr. Kraisintu. We must make some profit, however small. Producing antiretrovirals is an unknown as far as profits are concerned. Why risk it?

DR. KRISANA. It will be profitable. I promise you.

DIRECTOR LIKHIT. It's going to be complicated and it's going to be expensive.

DR. KRISANA. It will be profitable.

DIRECTOR LIKHIT. But we are profitable, now! Thanks to your excellent work here, we are making a profit. Your division has introduced nearly one hundred new GPO products since you started it. Look at this one (*points at a GPO product on the screen*)—this was a good one. And this one (*points at another*)—we sell over 400,000 doses per month. Take a holiday, Dr. Kraisintu. You work too hard, if you don't mind my saying so. I'm going on a short vacation myself this weekend. Your dedication is admirable but why not take a break? Nobody here works fifteen-hour days like you do.

DR. KRISANA. Director Likhit, I am certain producing antiretrovirals will be profitable. It can't help being profitable. There's an epidemic going on here in Thailand. That is why it will be profitable, unfortunately.

DIRECTOR LIKHIT. We are not a chemical company, Dr. Kraisintu. You know we cannot synthesize these AIDS medications ourselves. And surely you do not believe that the American pharmaceutical companies that make them will sell the raw materials to you?

DR. KRISANA. The large pharmaceutical companies do not make the chemicals themselves, either. They purchase them, in bulk, from general chemical suppliers.

The panda walks across stage reading a newspaper.

DR. KRISANA. (*Continues*) Then they press them into pills, and sell the pills for many times their cost to make. We can buy our ingredients from these same chemical companies.

DIRECTOR LIKHIT. This is not aspirin or ibuprofen we're talking about.

DR. KRISANA. I have already contacted a few chemical companies. I already have price estimates from Samchully in Korea and Ajinomoto in Japan.

DIRECTOR LIKHIT. Ajinomoto? I thought they made MSG.

The panda looks up when he hears "Ajinomoto," then exits.

DR. KRISANA. They do. They also make the antiretroviral drugs ddI and stavudine.

DIRECTOR LIKHIT. Dr. Kraisintu, do you know what a TRIPs agreement is?

DR. KRISANA. I think I do. But it does not really concern me.

DIRECTOR LIKHIT. Ah, but it does concern you. It concerns me. It concerns all of us here at the GPO. The agreement on Trade Related Aspects of Intellectual Property Rights. This is part of Thailand's ticket to the future. Not signing it is the mark of a third-world backwater of a country. Thailand has signed it—which is the mark of a first-world economy.

DR. KRISANA. These international patent agreements only protect the American pharmaceutical companies.

DIRECTOR LIKHIT. TRIPs agreements protect the patent rights of all companies, regardless of their country of origin. They are simply good business. You are on dangerous ground, Dr. Kraisintu. You are going to jeopardize our country's trade relations with the United States. Some countries have already seen severe sanctions imposed.

DR. KRISANA. I promise you we can continue to manufacture everything you mentioned plus antiretrovirals and turn a profit. Besides, once I succeed, it may be profitable outside of Thailand. AIDS has already spread to Cambodia, to Laos, beyond our borders. This epidemic does not respect national boundaries.

DIRECTOR LIKHIT. Who is going to trust antiretrovirals manufactured from an Asian source?

DR. KRISANA. What's wrong with an Asian source?

DIRECTOR LIKHIT. Besides, it's too dangerous.

DR. KRISANA. What?

DIRECTOR LIKHIT. It's dangerous. Dr. Kraisintu, we have over two thousand workers here at the GPO. I am not going to risk lives around a psychotoxic substance.

DR. KRISANA. It's not that toxic.

DIRECTOR LIKHIT. Honestly, do you think any staff here would be willing to take the risk?

DR. KRISANA. It's not that risky. And it only really concerns my own staff.

DIRECTOR LIKHIT. You think Thatsani, Chuchit, Kitiphan, and the rest will follow you?

DR. KRISANA. (*Pause*) They may take some convincing, but eventually—

DIRECTOR LIKHIT. I'm against it, and don't forget, you will still have the union to contend with, and I don't think they are going to like it any more than I do. Look, Dr. Kraisintu, we are—we are more than happy with everything you are doing now. There's no need to stir things up.

DR. KRISANA. I'd like to try.

DIRECTOR LIKHIT. To stir things up? Take a vacation, Dr. Kraisintu.

DR. KRISANA. You said that already, sir.

DIRECTOR LIKHIT. (*Very angry*) Fine! Have it your way. Quite frankly, I don't think you will be successful. I think that this will be a waste of both time and money. Now I have to be going. Is there anything else I can help you with?

DR. KRISANA. No. Thank you for taking the time to talk to me. I'm sure you're very busy. I won't take up any more of your time. Good afternoon, sir.

DIRECTOR LIKHIT. Good afternoon.

Dr. Krisana exits. Sound of a door slam.

DIRECTOR LIKHIT. (*He speaks to his secretary over an intercom.*) Call my chauffeur. I'm going to the airport. And, um . . . see if you can connect me to Brighton Miles.

Sound: Ticking stays up. In a hallway. A little reverberant.

Achara has been anxiously waiting to hear the results.

ACHARA. Did Director Likhit agree to help?

DR. KRISANA. Director Likhit has agreed to let me do it—but grudgingly. I think that Dr. Likhit is more concerned with profits than with patients. I don't think he'll be giving us much support. I'm going to miss Dr. Bhunbhu. Did you talk to Chuchit and the others?

ACHARA. Well, I—

DR. KRISANA. Did they agree to help? (*Achara is silent.*) What did they say?

ACHARA. They are waiting to speak with you.

Staff 1 (Kitiphan), Staff 2 (Chuchit), and Staff 3 (Thatsani) enter sheepishly.

DR. KRISANA. So this is how it is?

STAFF 2 (CHUCHIT). Even the dust from these chemicals is toxic. Think of the labor union—would they even allow it?

STAFF 1 (KITIPHAN). And the raw materials are very expensive.

STAFF 3 (THATSANI). The treatments are very complicated. Each patient must take two or three different kinds.

STAFF 1 (Kitiphan). How would we—

STAFF 2 (Chuchit). I heard that the dust can make you feel ill, and throw up.

STAFF 3 (Thatsani). Is the GPO ready for something like this?

STAFF 2 (Chuchit). Has the director approved this?

STAFF 1 (KITIPHAN). Could the Thai people afford them, even if we could make them?

STAFF 3 (Thatsani). This would be more complicated than anything we make now.

DR. KRISANA. But Thatsani, you remember antihistamines were difficult at first, but you eventually succeeded. Kitiphan, you helped me devise the correct formulation for several of our products. These were not easy tasks. What have you to say?

Staff 1 (Kitiphan) remains silent. He puts his head down.

DR. KRISANA. (*She is angry.*) Achara, get the building super.

ACHARA. Get the building super?

DR. KRISANA. Achara, do you need an ear cleaning? I said, get the building super.

ACHARA. What are you going to do?

DR. KRISANA. I'm going to empty out the storage room and start working on antiretrovirals.

ACHARA. Alone?!

THE OTHERS. Alone?

DR. KRISANA. Apparently.

A stagehand brings on her cleansuit; she puts it on.

ACHARA. But Dr. Krisana, you can't do it alone.

DR. KRISANA. Help me empty out the storage room.

ACHARA. Me?!

DR. KRISANA. Yes, you. Are you coming or not? (*She exits.*)

ACHARA. (*Rushing after her*) Yes, Dr. Krisana. (*All exit.*)

SCENE 10. MAKING THE PILL

Sound: Ticking bumps out and music bumps in. Music is slow, lonely, minimalist.

A lab table, on wheels, with equipment and chemicals, is brought on by a stagehand. On the table there should be a single-punch pill press, a small weighing scale, a half dozen chemical bottles, chemical spatulas, chemical weigh boats, other assorted lab supplies. Dr. Krisana enters in the black. She is wearing a cleansuit. Lights up. She begins to work on making pills. The exact activities she performs during the scene will depend on the exact lab equipment available for a production, but could/ should include weighing chemicals on the scale, mixing chemical powders from different bottles, pressing pills with the pill press, examining the pills, cutting the pills in half and examining the inside, crushing pills with a mortar and pestle, dissolving pills in a beaker of liquid. Dr. Krisana should work continuously throughout the scene. The scene can be paced with any variation of spacing between lines. The two "Date People" are dressed in black and say their lines from the edges of the stage.

DATE PERSON 1. Monday evening, 8 PM. September 16, 1991.
DATE PERSON 2. Sunday evening, 9:30 PM. November 6, 1991.

Live Feed Projection: A live camera feed shows the central portion of Dr. Krisana's "lab bench." The camera is located above Dr. Krisana's work area, and the live feed image is projected on the screen.

Achara enters with a bottle of AZT.

Projection: The chemical structure of AZT is projected behind her, following her. This image travels superimposed over the Live Feed.

Achara exits.

DATE PERSON 1. One hour, two hours, three hours, twelve hours.

DATE PERSON 2. 10 PM, 11 PM, 12 PM, 1:05 AM.

Achara enters again.

ACHARA. Dr. Krisana, you have a call from the Ministry of Health.

DR. KRISANA. Hold my calls.

Dr. Krisana works.

DATE PERSON 1. The pills won't bind.

DATE PERSON 2. The pills won't bind.

DATE PERSON 1. The pills won't bind.

DATE PERSON 2. The pills won't bind.

DATE PERSON 1. The pills fall apart.

DATE PERSON 2. The pills fall apart.

DATE PERSON 1. The pills fall apart.

DATE PERSON 2. The pills fall apart.

*Projection: The Bangkok skyline at dusk, very slowly fading into evening at
normal speed.*

 Dr. Krisana sits on a stool next to the bench. She is exhausted.

DATE PERSON 1 AND 2: Spring, Summer, Fall, Winter.

 Achara enters with tea.

DR. KRISANA. No tea in the clean room. You know that, Achara. (*She rises
and goes back to work at the bench.*)

DATE PERSON 1. Time passes.

DATE PERSON 2. Time passes.

DATE PERSON 1. Time passes.

DATE PERSON 2. Time passes.

ACHARA. Dr. Krisana, I was going to go home for the night. Do you need
anything else?

DR. KRISANA. (*Handing her a pill*) Look, Achara! It's an AZT tablet.

ACHARA. Oh, my God! Is it true? It's a miracle.

DR. KRISANA. (*Laughs*) It's not a miracle, Achara—it's just pharmacology. And look: I'm still alive! This is only the beginning. Full treatment requires taking three different drugs a day to stay alive— sometimes ten or twenty pills a day, depending on the drugs. But I think it may be possible to combine different drugs into one pill. I need these chemicals. (*She hands a list to Achara. Achara exits.*)

Projection: Skyline out and live feed up.

> *Director Likhit enters and looks at Dr. Krisana at work and then begins a slow cross, but keeps to the perimeter of the stage.*

> *Voice-over (VO) of Dr. Krisana and Achara talking, as Dr. Krisana keeps working and Achara brings her chemicals. The voice-over is not synchronized with any onstage action.*

DR. KRISANA, VO. Achara, I need a better binder—to hold the different chemicals together.

ACHARA, VO. Dr. Krisana, I've ordered the chemicals you asked for.
Achara re-enters with ddI.

Projection: The chemical structure of ddI is projected and travels from the top of the screen to the bottom of the screen.

DR. KRISANA, VO. Achara, they keep falling apart. There must be a better way to hold them together.

ACHARA, VO. Dr. Krisana, I've put all the papers you need to sign on your desk. It's very late. Don't you think it's time for you to go home?

DR. KRISANA, VO. I'm fine, Achara.

ACHARA, VO. But you need to sleep.

DR. KRISANA, VO. I'm fine Achara. Don't be a pest.

ACHARA, VO. I will see you first thing in the morning. First thing.

DR. KRISANA, VO. Achara, this combination still falls apart too easily. Can you look up some pressure conversion constants for me?
Director Likhit, on the edge of the stage, makes a phone call to a BMP executive.

DIRECTOR LIKHIT. Hello. Brighton Miles?

BMP 6. (*On the edge of the stage*) Ah, Dr. Likhit, I've been expecting your call.

DR. KRISANA, VO. Achara, maybe Dr. Likhit and the others are right. Maybe this is asking too much.

Projection: The live feed is wiped out and is replaced by the Bangkok skyline.

Achara enters on the side with Staff 1 (Kitiphan), Staff 2 (Chuchit), and Staff 3 (Thatsani). Dr. Krisana continues to work inside her "room."

STAFF 1 (Kitiphan). What do you mean, one pill?

ACHARA. That's what she said.

STAFF 1 (KITIPHAN). All three drugs in one pill? In one tablet?

ACHARA. Yes, yes, that's what she said. Why? What is wrong?

STAFF 1 (KITIPHAN). Nothing is wrong. It's just . . . It's just that . . .

STAFF 3 (THATSANI). It's unprecedented.

STAFF 1 (Kitiphan). It's never been done before.

ACHARA. That's good, right?

STAFF 1 (KITIPHAN). I ah . . . could you tell her that I would like to speak to her?

ACHARA. Yes. Yes, of course. Just a moment.
Achara enters Dr. Krisana's room and talks to her. Staff 1 (Kitiphan), Staff 2 (Chuchit), and Staff 3 (Thatsani) are animatedly discussing, almost arguing. Dr. Krisana and Achara come out.

DR. KRISANA. Kitiphan.

STAFF 1 (KITIPHAN). Is it true? You've combined stavudine, lamivudine, and nevirapine into a single pill?

DR. KRISANA. Take a look. I'm thinking of calling it a triple cocktail.

Dr. Krisana hands him a single pill. He holds it up to look at it.

STAFF 1 (Kitiphan). But how do you hold it together?

DR. KRISANA. The binder is a carageenan.

STAFF 1 (Kitiphan). From red seaweed.

DR. KRISANA. Yes.

STAFF 1 (Kitiphan). You have always been fond of the carageenans.

DR. KRISANA. What can I say? I grew up on an island. I like seaweed.

STAFF 1 (KITIPHAN). This is unprecedented.

DR. KRISANA. It's not finished yet. The pills are still too fragile, and too large. But, I think I can do it without the binder, by direct compression with only the three drugs—in order to reduce the size of the tablet.

STAFF 1 (Kitiphan). Dr. Kraisintu. I would very much like . . . I would like your permission to . . . obtain a cleansuit . . . and to assist you in your current research.

DR. KRISANA. That would make me very happy, Kitiphan.

ACHARA. (*Holds out a packaged cleansuit, Dr. Krisana and Staff 1 (Kitiphan) both look surprised*) I picked one up from inside the room just now, just in case.

Staff 1 (Kitiphan) takes the cleansuit from Achara.

Fade to black.

SCENE 11. MEET TIDO

Sound: Ticking bumps in.

Projection: Text "Several months later".

Projection: Outline of Africa map (as before), only now with AIDS prevalence distribution during late 1990s or early 2000 fading in.

DR. KRISANA. Achara, make an appointment for me with Director Likhit.
Director Likhit enters as Dr. Krisana is speaking.
DIRECTOR LIKHIT. No appointment necessary. How are you Dr. Kraisintu?
DR. KRISANA. The triple-drug cocktail is not selling.
DIRECTOR LIKHIT. Yes, I know.
DR. KRISANA. None of my antiretrovirals are selling.
DIRECTOR LIKHIT. Yes. I know.
During this conversation, Tido enters. He appears lost. He is wandering around in some other part of the building.
DR. KRISANA. I thought perhaps if the GPO were to advertise the availability of the new antiretrovirals more vigorously . . .
DIRECTOR LIKHIT. Things are not always as straightforward as they seem, Dr. Kraisintu.
DR. KRISANA. I took the liberty of purchasing some advertisements of my own, in a few of the local magazines and newspapers. Just in the past few days.
DIRECTOR LIKHIT. That is very industrious of you, Dr. Kraisintu, but perhaps in the future you should clear such activities with me first. The GPO should not appear to consist of a band of wild elephants.
DR. KRISANA. I apologize, Director, it's just that I still believe that—
DIRECTOR LIKHIT. As scientists, we are not paid to deal in beliefs, Dr. Kraisintu. We deal in the facts. Perhaps it is time for you to face them.

DR. KRISANA. Yes, Director.

Director Likhit leaves. During the following lines Tido comes up behind Dr. Krisana. Achara sees him and tries to motion to Dr. Krisana that there is someone behind her (clears her throat, points, etc.). Achara does this several times, louder and louder, before Dr. Krisana finally notices.

DR. KRISANA. Perhaps Director Likhit is right, Achara, but I just don't understand how. Thailand is in dire need of antiretrovirals—so why is no one buying them? If I were a suspicious person . . . but I don't want to think about such possibilities. I don't want to hurt the GPO. Perhaps I—what in the world are you doing, Achara?

ACHARA. I think there is someone here to see you.

DR. KRISANA. Oh, hello.

TIDO. Hello. Are you Dr. Kraisintu?

DR. KRISANA. Yes.

TIDO. My name is Tido von Schoen-Angerer.

ACHARA. That's quite a mouthful.

DR. KRISANA. (*She looks at Achara reproachfully.*) What can we do for you?

TIDO. I am with Doctors Without Borders here in Thailand. I've been told that someone here at the GPO has developed a drug cocktail for HIV treatment that only has to be taken twice a day. However, I can't get any more information. Several people mentioned your name. I'm very sorry if I am bothering you.

DR. KRISANA. Oh my goodness, no, no—I mean, yes, I mean, yes, we have the triple cocktail.

TIDO. It's true, then? Three drugs in one pill?

DR. KRISANA. Yes, yes.

TIDO. That's absolutely marvelous.

DR. KRISANA. Would you like to see how it is made?

TIDO. Why—yes, I would. I'd also like to discuss the possibility of purchasing a year's supply for approximately five thousand patients.

Dr. Krisana goes up to him and hugs him.

DR. KRISANA. Oh! You must be an angel!

TIDO. Hardly.

DR. KRISANA. Come, let me show you how we make them.

As they begin to exit, Staff 1 (Kitiphan) rushes in and approaches them.

DR. KRISANA. Kitiphan! This is Dr. von Schoen-Angerer. (*She mispronounces it, and laughs.*) I'm sorry, I didn't mean to—.

TIDO. (*Laughing*) Von Schoen-Angerer. Please, please call me Tido.

DR. KRISANA. Tido, this is my associate Kitiphan, one of my senior scientists. Kitiphan, you look like you've seen a ghost. What's wrong?

STAFF 1 (Kitiphan). Then you haven't heard. Director Likhit just told me that we are going to be visited by executives from Brighton Miles Pharmaceuticals—from America—the ones who own the patents on two of the generic antiretrovirals you have made.

DR. KRISANA. Director Likhit just told you this?

STAFF 1 (KITIPHAN). Yes.

DR. KRISANA. Well, well, no need to panic. We just have to make sure we are prepared with the proper facts. When are these representatives coming?

STAFF 1 (Kitiphan). Tomorrow.

DR. KRISANA. (*Shouting*) Tomorrow!

STAFF 1 (Kitiphan). There's going to be trouble.

Sound: Ticking bumps out.

SCENE 12. HIGH NOON

Sound: Music starts immediately after Staff 1 (Kitiphan) says "Tomorrow."

Tido, Achara, and Staff 1 (Kitiphan) exit. BMP 1–6 enter.

Projection: Africa is still on the screen, but it is now replaced by a structure of didanosine. This stays on until Dr. Krisana says "reverse transcriptase," at which time the structure of HIV reverse transcriptase appears. After Dr. Krisana's monologue, the structure of HIV reverse transcriptase fades, then viruses, smaller versions of the giant virus shown earlier, begin multiplying on the screen, until they fill the screen and start overlapping each other.

DR. KRISANA. (*She speaks directly to the audience.*) Look at this chemical. What do you see? (*She holds up a molecular model of ddI.*) This is ddI. It is a nucleotide analog. It looks complicated, but it's not. Your average high school student today has memorized chemical structures similar to this. It is almost identical to one of the normal building blocks of DNA, with one important exception: it's poison to the HIV virus. In order to reproduce itself, the HIV virus requires a protein called HIV reverse transcriptase.

Projection: HIV reverse transcriptase.

DR. KRISANA. You can think of HIV reverse transcriptase as a Xerox machine. After all, it's a protein that copies nucleic acids. ddI is the wrong brand of transparency for this Xerox machine. It jams up the whole works. Imagine putting peanut butter in your Xerox machine. The virus can't survive if it can't reproduce itself. That's how ddI stops the virus.

BMP 2. We know the chemistry.

BMP 3. Very well, we know it very well.

BMP 4. I think you should put that chemical down.

DR. KRISANA. Why should I put this down?

BMP 4. (*Politely*) Because you don't own it.

DR. KRISANA. (*Pause*) Neither do you.

BMP 2. Yes, I'm afraid we do.

BMP 3. We own the patent on ddI, and on stavudine, both of which we understand you are attempting to manufacture here in Thailand.

DR. KRISANA. There is no patent on these drugs in Thailand.

BMP 4. Oh, I think you're wrong about that. Especially about ddI.

BMP 5. (*Green dots slowly fade up on BMP 5 as the scene progresses.*) Wrong, wrong, wrong.

BMP 6. We filed for the patent for ddI almost two years ago.

DR. KRISANA. There is no patent on ddI in Thailand.

BMP 6. (*To BMP 4*) You were the one who signed the OM481, correct?

BMP 4. (*To BMP 6*) Of course, I remember it well. I also filed the IM220 and USPTO release.

BMP 6. (*To BMP 4*) Yes, certainly, certainly, you would have to. I'm trying to remember seeing them cross my desk.

BMP 4. (*To BMP 6*) That was the summer you had the affair with my secretary.

BMP 6. (*To BMP 4*) Oh yes! Of course! Now I remember. I remember it clearly. Ah, I can see the forms, right there on the desk behind what's-her-name's head.

BMP 4. (*Almost to self*) She was a good secretary. Good ole what's-her-name.

BMP 6. (*To Dr. Krisana*) So, yes, I'm afraid we do own the patent, even in Thailand.

DR. KRISANA. It was invented at the National Institutes of Health, in the U.S.

BMP 3. Yes, yes, of course, and they patented it, and sold the patent to us—that's the way patent law works, in case you don't know.

BMP 1. It protects the investment.

BMP 2. So that other people will invent things. Who would invent anything, if they couldn't watch their investment grow and grow?

BMP 1. No one! Who would invent new drugs?

BMP 3. Who would invest in new therapies, if they didn't think they could get a return, a reward for their effort?

BMP 2. A doggie bone.

BMP 3. (*Barks twice*).

BMP 2. (*Barks*).

BMP 6. (*Barks*).

BMP 4. (*Barks*).

BMP 1. (*Barks*).

BMP 4. We were wondering how familiar you are with international patent law?

DR. KRISANA. But people are dying.

BMP 1. Yes, yes, of course people are dying. And it's terrible. It's a crime. People are dying all the time. And that's why we need to insure that innovation and invention are duly rewarded. Then we can eventually eradicate all disease. But if we gave drugs away . . .

BMP 2. We can't give drugs away.

BMP 3. Certainly not. That's a no-brainer.

BMP 4. What a ridiculous notion. The pharmaceutical industry as we know it would cease to exist.

BMP 5. Hilarious. (*Laughs for a long time*) No, no, no way.

BMP 1. Of course, I'm only posing a hypothetical illustration. If we gave drugs away, who would invent new drugs? There would be no incentive.

BMP 6. No one would invent new drugs.

BMP 2. No one.

BMP 3. Not a soul. Nada.

BMP 4. No one in their right mind, anyway.

BMP 3. (*Barks twice*).

BMP 1. (*Barks*).

BMP 6. (*Barks*).

BMP 5. Would you please stop doing that? My head already hurts.

BMP 3. Uh oh, looks like somebody can't hold their liquor.

DR. KRISANA. The fact that people are dying today from a treatable disease is not a hypothetical situation. Children are—

BMP 1. Ah, the children.

BMP 3. The children!

BMP 2. The children.

BMP 6. The children.

BMP 4. Always the children. (*To BMP 2*) Breath mint?

BMP 2. No, thanks. You can't fight the dying children.

BMP 1. There's no way.

BMP 5. It just shuts off all useful discourse.

BMP 2. It's grandstanding, plain and simple. How do you trump a dying child?

BMP 1. You can't.

BMP 3. You can't.

BMP 6. You can't.

BMP 4. It just shuts down the conversation every time.

BMP 2. Why, if I had a nickel for every dying child . . .

BMP 1. You'd be rich my friend, you'd be rich.

    All BMPs laugh.

BMP 5. Listen, lady . . .

BMP 1. She's a doctor.

BMP 5. Excuse me?

BMP 1. She's a doctor. A Ph.D. Show some respect, you piece of shit.

BMP 5. I'm sorry, I'm a bit hungover. (*He puts his head in his hands.*)

BMP 1. Dr. Kriteersion.

DR. KRISANA. Kraisintu.

BMP 1. Gesundheit. The point is, we've come here today as a courtesy call. We're all in this fight together. Against this terrible disease.

BMP 2. This plague.

BMP 3. This pestilence.

BMP 4. (*To BMP 3*) What is the market here, anyway?

BMP 3. I don't know. What country are we in again?

DR. KRISANA. The "market," as you call it, is nearly 400,000 dying human beings. There are nearly 400,000 people in Thailand dying of AIDS right now because they cannot afford your medications. Almost a quarter of those are children—babies. Babies born with HIV. How can you, in good conscience, not want to save the babies?

BMP 2. Oh, now who's the Gloomy Gus?

BMP 5. (*He had his head down for a while, but now looks up and laughs.*) Did she just say "shave the babies"?

BMP 1. No! No, she did not say "shave the babies," you stupid fuck! If you hadn't spent all night drinking in a brothel you might be able to keep up with the program here.

BMP 3. (*Attempts to calm the situation*) Listen, 400,000 with HIV—that's 400,000 people who could be helped by our medications. As long as nobody screws everything up by giving it away or something. Not that we're saying you're doing anything wrong.

BMP 2. International patent law is very complicated.

DR. KRISANA. There is no patent on ddI in Thailand.

BMP 3. TRIPs legislation is VERY complicated. You really need to be a lawyer to understand it.

BMP 4. Yes, so we would never tell you that you are doing anything wrong.

BMP 5. Oh no, that's not our place. We would never directly tell you that you are violating our patent.

BMP 6. We'd never tell you that such violations could result in jail time.

BMP 2. Trade sanctions.

BMP 3. Embargoes.

BMP 4. International blacklisting.

BMP 5. Revocation of the license to practice medicine.

BMP 1. (*Slaps BMP 5*) I told you she's a Ph.D., she's not an M.D.

BMP 5. Well, whatever. We'd never tell her that anyway, even if she was.

BMP 1. Listen, Dr. Kolinstu.

DR. KRISANA. Kraisintu.

BMP 1. Yes, yes, of course. What we want you to know is that we too, all of us, feel your pain and urgency in this matter, and respect your lack of understanding of the complexities involved, and the need for a coherent and encompassing global vision. And we want you to know that we've come here as friends. And friends, true friends, are honest with one another. Friends don't let friends drive drunk. When they see that a friend might harm themselves, they take the keys away from that friend, in a gesture of friendship. (*He takes the chemical model of ddI from her.*) I'm sure you understand.

BMP 2. I'm hungry. Is anybody hungry?

BMP 3. I'm starving.

BMP 4. Second that.

BMP 2. *Pad thai?*

BMP 4. Second that.

BMP 1. Well, I think we have to be going, Dr. Kraisinshun. (*He puts his hands together in a distorted Thai gesture of leave-taking.*) I want to thank you for your time, and your consideration in this matter. I can see that you're one tough cookie.

DR. KRISANA. (*She approaches BMP 1*) Yes, I am. You're right. I am. (*She reaches for the ddI chemical model to take it back, but BMP 1 tosses it to a colleague, who exits with it.*)
BMP 4, 5, 6, and Dr. Krisana exit.

SCENE 13. BMP ON THE WARPATH

Sound: Low, repetitive music with building tension.

Projection: Text "From 5 to 100 milligrams per dose" crosses the screen from stage right to stage left and then goes out.

BMP 1 takes out a phone and dials.

GIRL FROM COMMERCIAL. (*Speaks in Japanese*) Moshi, moshi, Ajinomoto Seiyaku.

BMP 1. (*Annoyed*) Uh, yes, hello, do you speak English?

GIRL. Ajinomoto Chemical, how may I help you?

BMP 1. I'd like to speak with Hiro Takeda.

GIRL. May I ask who is calling, sir?

BMP 1. Tell him Brighton Miles Pharmaceuticals is calling.

GIRL. One moment, sir (*short pause*).

PANDA. (*Enters and sits*) Hiro here. Konnichiwa.

BMP 1. Hiro. This is Robert. Konnichiwa, you SOB!

PANDA. Ah, Robert-san. It is always a pleasure to speak to you. What can I do for you today?

BMP 1. Hiro, Hiro, Hiro. It's come to our attention that Ajinomoto has been selling ddI to customers other than our company.

PANDA. Hai?

BMP 1. That's naughty, naughty, you know.

PANDA. Naughty? Excuse me? I don't quite understand.

BMP 1. Well, Hiro, perhaps you'll understand this: Brighton Miles will be needing all the ddI you can produce there at Ajinomoto. All of it, you understand? You cannot make enough to sell it to any other customers. It's simply not possible, is it? Do you understand?

PANDA. Hai. You are always right Robert-san. Absolutely right. I am deeply sorry that we have made this unpardonable mistake. And so will you be making many more doses then, Robert-san?

BMP 1. Will we be making many more doses? (*Laughs*) I like you Hiro. You're a funny guy. But listen, Ajinomoto's production subcontract with Brighton is up for renewal in a couple of months, and I would hate to see any problems with that.

PANDA. I understand, Robert-san. Thank you for correcting our mistake.

BMP 1. Good, good. Sayonara, Hiro.

PANDA. Sayonara.

Projection: Text "5 TO 100 MILLIGRAMS PER DOSE" *appears in horizontal scroll from off left of screen to screen center and stops while rest of text of patent appears above and below it.*

BMP 2 is on the phone, BMP 3 is next to him/her.

BMP 2. Hi, Rosey. This is Jack(ie). I need to talk to someone in Legal. (*Pause*) Hello, who is this? Oh, great. Listen, what's the status on the ddI patent in Thailand? (*Pause*) Really? I thought it was settled. What's the problem? What line? It's being held up because of a single line?

BMP 3. (*To BMP 2*) What line? And why is this line so important?

BMP 2. (*To BMP 3*) How do I know? (*Into phone*) Un huh, uh huh. (*To BMP 3*) The line is "5 to 100 milligrams per dose."

BMP 3. And so?

BMP 2. (*To BMP 3*) Wait. (*Into phone*) Uh huh, uh huh. Hold on. (*To BMP 3*) Because the GPO, this woman, is planning to make tablets with 100 milligrams and 300 milligrams.

BMP 3. (*Slowly, thinking it through*) So unless we take that line out of the patent, they can perfectly legally make any size tablet they want outside of the 5 to 100 milligram range?

BMP 2. Bingo, Einstein.

BMP 3. So what do we do?

BMP 2. I think some people at the GPO know which side of their bread is buttered. Some people here know how to avoid tripping over TRIPs, if you know what I mean. *(BMP 3 laughs or snorts a bit too cloyingly at each of BMP 2's lame jokes, which only annoys BMP 2.)*

BMP 2. *(Continues)* Some people here understand pressure points, as in acupressure *(BMP 2 presses on BMP 3 with two fingers until BMP 3 yelps)*. *(Speaking to BMP 3 with an accent)* I'm-a da World Trade-a Organization, an I'm-a gonna make you an offa ya can't refuse. *(Returning to speaking on the phone)* Hey, I'm back. Listen, delete the line. *(Pause)* Yes, on my authority. *(Pause)* I don't care if the king of Thailand himself already approved it. Delete the fucking line. And ram this thing through ASAP. Do you understand me?

Sound: Thunder and rain with ticking underneath.

Projection: Only the line "5 TO 100 MILLIGRAMS PER DOSE" *fades out.*

SCENE 14. TIDO & DR. KRISANA FIGHT BACK

Sound: Raining throughout with ticking underneath.

Tido slaps some papers down on Dr. Krisana's desk. He is angry.

TIDO. Look, look, right there. That's where they deleted the line. Right there.

DR. KRISANA. Tido, I know. Do you know how many times I've read through this patent?

TIDO. I'm sorry, Krisana, I'm just . . .

DR. KRISANA. I don't understand why they didn't also go after stavudine. They have the U.S. patent on that, too.

TIDO. But you can still make the triple-drug cocktail, right?

DR. KRISANA. Well, yes, yes—as long as they don't somehow cut off my supply of stavudine, too. ddI is not in the cocktail, but ddI is important, too. We're trying to develop other combination pills with ddI in them now.

TIDO. So this cuts off treatment options.

DR. KRISANA. Many. And research options, new development. Tido, is there anything you can do? Doctors Without Borders is an international organization. Perhaps we can set up manufacture in Cambodia or Laos?

TIDO. We don't have the infrastructure for something like that. And it's ridiculous—it's ridiculous that we should have to consider such a thing.

ACHARA. *(Almost growling)* It's criminal. They're criminals.

TIDO. *(Amused at Achara's outburst)* Morally, yes. Legally, unfortunately, no. In fact, if we go ahead with manufacture of pills with ddI in them, we'll be the criminals. But, you know . . . *(pause)*.

DR. KRISANA. Tido, what are you thinking?

TIDO. What if we sue Brighton Miles Pharmaceuticals?

DR. KRISANA. Us? Sue them?

TIDO. Yes. They removed the line "from 5 to 100 milligrams" from the Thai patent after it was approved by parliament, but before it was approved by the Thai Office of Intellectual Property. We sue them for improper implementation of international patent approval.

DR. KRISANA. But there is no official procedure for international patent approval. It hasn't been written.

TIDO. Exactly.

DR. KRISANA. And while the patent is in appeal, can I manufacture ddI?

TIDO. I think, technically, yes—as long as you can get someone to sell you raw materials. And, if your buyers don't balk at a pending lawsuit. At least on that end, I'm fairly confident that Doctors Without Borders won't have a problem buying it.

DR. KRISANA. Achara, get Ajinomoto on the phone. And if they still won't sell raw materials to me, I'll need a list of all chemical companies worldwide that make any type of DNA or RNA nucleotide. If they make one, they can make another.

ACHARA. Yes, Dr. Krisana, right away. (*She exits.*)

DR. KRISANA. (*To Tido*) So, how do we file this lawsuit?

TIDO. You don't file anything. You cannot be directly involved in this. This is for me, and for Doctors Without Borders. It's best if you just watch it on the news.

DR. KRISANA. So what do I do?

TIDO. Pray that the companies that own the other chemicals in your pills continue to look the other way. (*He sighs.*) Are you hungry? I am starving. How about some *pad thai*? My treat. (*They exit.*)

Sound: Cross bump from rain to channel switch.

SCENE 15. BBC 3

Projection: Simulated BBC newscast.

SELENA SCOTT. Good evening. This is the BBC World Service for December 22, 1999, and I'm Selena Scott. Representatives of the estimated half million Thais infected with HIV set up camp outside Thailand's Health Ministry on Wednesday to demand that the government break a U.S. drug firm's monopoly on an AIDS drug. About one hundred protesters, wearing yellow T-shirts, called on the government to issue a compulsory license to allow cheap local production of drugs produced and marketed by U.S. drug giant Brighton Miles Pharmaceuticals. Protesters are receiving support from Doctors Without Borders, the France-based international organization that won this year's Nobel Peace Prize. Protesters and Doctors Without Borders have erected tents, sleeping and cooking areas, and have vowed to continue their protests around the clock for at least a week.
Screen goes to static.

OPTIONAL INTERMISSION POINT FOR A TWO-ACT PRODUCTION

The pace of the subsequent scenes can be decidedly slower and more relaxed than the pace of the preceding scenes. Three years have passed.

SCENE 16. BARCELONA WORLD AIDS CONFERENCE

Sound: Auditorium ambience fades up. Reverb in large hall, occasional cough in audience, perhaps.

Projection: "WORLD AIDS CONFERENCE 2002 BARCELONA" with the conference logo.

Voice-over: Woman's voice, soothing, atmospheric, repeats multiple times, in several of the official languages of the United Nations: English, Spanish, French, Chinese, Russian, and Arabic, "Welcome to the 2002 World AIDS Conference. Welcome to Barcelona."

Conferees enter and sit and are engaged in conversation, or reading, or eating, until the Session Chair gets their attention. Tido enters at some point and watches from the back.

SESSION CHAIR. I think it's time to start this session. Welcome. Our first speaker this afternoon is, um, Dr. Krisana Kraisintu, Head of Research and Development for the Thai Government Pharmaceutical Organization.

DR. KRISANA. Fellow researchers, pharmaceutical scientists, and respected physicians. Over the past several years, we have had many successes in HIV treatment and prevention in Thailand. The number of new HIV cases in Thailand has fallen to 21,000 this year, from a high of 140,000 in 1991. The GPO, the Thai Government Pharmaceutical Organization, now produces four generic anti-HIV reverse transcriptase inhibitors for our own population. AZT . . .

Projection: Structure of AZT and a bottle of pills.

DR. KRISANA. . . . stavudine . . .

Projection: Structure of stavudine.

DR. KRISANA. . . . lamivudine . . .

Projection: Structure of lamivudine.

DR. KRISANA. . . . and nevirapine.

Projection: Structure of nevirapine.

DR. KRISANA. But today I want to introduce to you a new formulation, which I have named GPO-VIR. GPO-VIR is a single tablet containing these three antiretrovirals: stavudine, lamivudine, and nevirapine.

Projection: A movie plays showing the three chemicals rotating and then getting smaller and "dissolving" into a single, large white tablet.

SESSION CHAIR. I'm sorry, but I think you mistakenly said that you combined three HIV drugs into the same tablet.
DR. KRISANA. Yes, yes, I did say that. This formulation will increase patient compliance—especially among children, the poor, and the illiterate, who will now need only to take two tablets each day to treat their infection. After several years in development, the GPO produced an initial batch of 120,000 pills of GPO-VIR in March of this year. They are being sold at GPO retail pharmacies for the equivalent of 92 cents, U.S., per day, making this the lowest-priced AIDS treatment in the world.
Many conferees raise their hands for questions. Several nearly shout "Dr. Kraisintu?"

CONFEREE 1. Dr. Kraisintu?

DR. KRISANA. Yes?

CONFEREE 1. Aren't these three drugs in your cocktail patented by different companies?

DR. KRISANA. I believe so, yes.

CONFEREE 1. You believe so? But you don't know?

DR. KRISANA. I try not to concern myself with this kind of information. I consult the treatment guides to see what antiretrovirals can be successfully combined.

CONFEREE 1. But what about TRIPs and the World Trade Organization—this must figure in your work?

DR. KRISANA. There have been certain challenges, yes. Some companies have supported our efforts. Others have not. We have been involved in a lawsuit regarding the drug ddI for several years now. During this time we have had no access to ddI. None whatsoever. No one in the world will sell it to us. However, I developed the three-drug cocktail I am presenting to you today with stavudine, lamivudine, and nevirapine—but with no ddI. It is very effective with this drug combination. I believe this new formulation will revolutionize treatment in Thailand.

CONFEREE 2. Dr. Kraisintu? What will you do when Thai patients begin developing drug resistance to these particular antiretrovirals? Isn't this a little risky?

CONFEREE 3. Yes, how can you insure compliance? If people don't take their pills correctly, you could create widespread resistance to all three drugs.

CONFEREE 4. Do you have a distribution plan?

DR. KRISANA. If you allow such concerns to stop you from acting, then nothing will get done, and people will die. Lots of people have already died. I can make these tablets. If people take them, they will live longer. Where is the problem?

CONFEREE 4. Please don't misinterpret. I have been following your work in Thailand. This is a wonderful achievement, something that should have been done years ago, when multi-drug treatment began.

DR. KRISANA. Yes, yes, exactly.

CONFEREE 4. But it is important to think about the future, about control of resistance, about proper distribution among populations with histories of poor compliance. Critics of your work have said that you will eventually induce drug-resistant strains of HIV in Thailand.

DR. KRISANA. I would ask these critics if they would rather see people die now because they might become resistant later? For years now I have been told that what I am doing is wrong. That I am violating international patents. That I cannot combine drugs from different companies into the same tablet. That my formulations will induce resistance to HIV. That I have personally caused trade sanctions against my country. The Thai people are— (*she suddenly stops and turns to the side. She is crying, but it is not immediately obvious.*) I'm sorry, just a moment. (*Short pause, then she collects herself and continues*) The Thai people are dying. We still cannot produce enough for our own population. The GPO has initiated plans to scale up production dramatically over the next several years.

CONFEREE 4. I'm sorry, I am only asking—what will you do next?

DR. KRISANA. What will I do next? What will I do next? (*Pause*) I will resign.

CONFEREE 4. Excuse me?

CONFEREE 1. What?

SESSION CHAIR. Pardon?

DR. KRISANA. Effective immediately upon my return to Bangkok, I will be resigning my position at the GPO, and I will be leaving my home country of Thailand.

Blackout.

SCENE 17. ON SAMUI II (SHADOW PLAY)

Sound: Ambient tropics. Sound of a single horse sauntering along on a dirty road. Quiet music, as in Scene I, but more menacing, more foreboding.

Projection: Digital animation of coconut palms on the island of Samui. Young Krisana and her grandmother are walking. The scenery is moving.

GRANDMOTHER. Krisana, will you ride with your father again today to see his patients in the villages?

YOUNG KRISANA. I love to ride with him on his visits. He has so many patients.

GRANDMOTHER. Yes. He is the only doctor on the island. We all need to help the world in some way.

YOUNG KRISANA. But, today I'd like to stay with you, Grandmother.

GRANDMOTHER. I'd like that very much.

YOUNG KRISANA. Grandmother, may I ask you a question?

GRANDMOTHER. Of course, Krisana, you can ask me anything.

YOUNG KRISANA. Why did you free your slaves?

GRANDMOTHER. Perhaps a better question to ask me is: why did I ever have slaves to begin with?

YOUNG KRISANA. I don't understand.

GRANDMOTHER. The world is always changing, little one. What once seemed good and true is perhaps not so good and true after all. We must respect all living beings, Krisana. I have spent much of my life learning how to do that, and I still have much to learn.

YOUNG KRISANA. Grandmother? May I ask you another question?

GRANDMOTHER. Goodness, child, of course, of course. I told you—always.

YOUNG KRISANA. Grandmother, should I leave Thailand, and move to Africa?

GRANDMOTHER. Excuse me, what? What did you say?

64

YOUNG KRISANA. The Thai Health Ministry has backed away from its promise of pharmaceutical tech transfer to Africa, and I wanted to know, do you think that I should leave Thailand and continue my work in Africa?

GRANDMOTHER. Goodness, child, what in the world are you talking about?

Sound: Bumps out and ambient room sound fades up.

SCENE 18. HEALTH MINISTER

Projection: Text "Thai Ministry of Health". Logo fills the screen.

> *Dr. Krisana enters. Two of the health minister's staff alternately step out and speak to Dr. Krisana as she is waiting. They tell her "The minister will see you now" several times, with long awkward pauses in between. Finally, Health Minister arrives.*

HEALTH MINISTER. (*Enters, unpacks his case at his desk for a while before speaking*) Dr. Kraisintu, please sit.

DR. KRISANA. Minister, thank you for seeing me. I won't take up much of your time. I simply wanted to know, when do you think we will go to Africa again?

HEALTH MINISTER. Ah, Dr. Kraisintu . . . Krisana. It is so good to see you. When I saw your name among my appointments today I must say I certainly smiled to myself. Now, I'm sorry, what did you ask me?

DR. KRISANA. I wanted to know when we would go to Africa again, to begin tech transfer.

HEALTH MINISTER. Well, I'm not sure that we will be going to Africa again, Krisana. That was three years ago when we announced that . . . 1999 to be exact.

DR. KRISANA. But we promised to help them make antiretrovirals. You spoke at the World Health Organization.

HEALTH MINISTER. Yes, and wasn't it wonderful? A seminal instant in history. For a moment all the world had its eyes on Thailand—and for biotechnology! I have heard that your HIV medications have become the most profitable products in the GPO. You should be very proud, Krisana.

DR. KRISANA. Thank you, Minister, but we must begin preparations for the technology transfer. There is a lot of information I can put in an instruction manual. However, there is much that must be demonstrated hands-on, one on one. There is an art to making pills, as well as a science.

HEALTH MINISTER. I applaud your enthusiasm, Krisana, and your tremendous accomplishments and contributions to our country, but Africa is no longer a priority for us.

DR. KRISANA. But you promised to help them. I promised to help them— Zimbabwe, Nigeria, Ghana. We reached out our hands to them. You signed a letter of agreement. They are all waiting for us.

HEALTH MINISTER. The moment has passed, Krisana. There are other priorities now. I see Thailand becoming a biotechnological giant, and I see you as a part of that future. Dr. Likhit has informed me that you tendered your resignation to him, but I believe he was correct in not accepting it.

DR. KRISANA. I resigned because he, too, refused to honor our promises in Africa. I have come here to appeal to you. We are developing adequate antiretroviral production in Thailand now. Much of it is free to our people, thanks to you and the Health Ministry. But, the people of Africa are dying. The people of Eritrea, Zimbabwe, Tanzania. We have the ability to help them. Unless we move forward on the promises we made to these countries, I see no reason to remain at the GPO.

HEALTH MINISTER. A first-world country has different health priorities, Krisana—you know that. Once the bane of tropical and sexually transmitted diseases are tamed, then the more complicated problems of cancer and heart disease can begin to be addressed.

DR. KRISANA. The people of Africa don't live long enough to get such diseases.

HEALTH MINISTER. Exactly, exactly, Krisana, but as Thailand moves into the future, we will need to more directly address these problems.

DR. KRISANA. You promised we would help them. I don't understand. You promised them me. I gave them my word that I would help.

HEALTH MINISTER. That moment has passed, Krisana. Let it go.

DR. KRISANA. I gave them my word. I gave them my promise. I cannot forget that.

HEALTH MINISTER. (*He goes over to her.*) I'm sorry, Krisana, but unless you plan on doing it all by yourself, you will just have to let it pass and move on to other priorities. I'm sure you understand. This is the way the world works, Krisana. We have to deal with the reality of the present moment. Krisana, listen to me. You speak the language of science. I speak the language of policy and politics. Together we make a team that will bring Thailand to the forefront of the world, as never before. You will come around to my way of thinking. It's only logical. Think of it. Think of the prestige. The prestige you will gain. It will be ten times what you have already achieved. I promise you. The sky's the limit. (*Pause. He returns to his desk.*) Good day, Krisana.

    As Dr. Krisana is exiting the health minister's office, her cell phone rings. The ambient sound goes out. Dr. Krisana answers the phone. Gebbers enters and speaks in German over the phone.

GEBBERS. Hallo. Mein Name ist Horst Gebbers, und wer sind Sie?
(*Translation: My name is Horst Gebbers, and who are you?*)

DR. KRISANA. (*Into the phone*) I'm sorry, I don't understand.

GEBBERS. Hallo, ist dort Thailand? Ich versuche Thailand zu erreichen!
(*Translation: Hello, is this Thailand? I'm trying to reach Thailand.*)

DR. KRISANA. Thailand? Yes! This is Thailand. I'm sorry, I don't speak your language.

GEBBERS. Dirk! Dirk!

    Dirk enters. Gebbers passes the phone off to Dirk.

DIRK. (*Speaking in English, but with a thick, German accent*) Hello. My name is Dirk Gebbers. I am calling on behalf of my father who would like to speak to a Dr. Krisana Kraisintu.

DR. KRISANA. I am Krisana Kraisintu.

DIRK. Excellent. Hello. We have read about your work in an article in *Der Spiegel*, the German magazine.

DR. KRISANA. Yes, that was a very flattering article.

DIRK. Our quinine factory was profiled in the same issue. Perhaps you saw our article?

DR. KRISANA. I'm afraid that I didn't—

DIRK. Doesn't matter. My father would very much like to meet you. He has a business proposition he would like to discuss. Can we bring you to our facility—at our expense, of course?

DR. KRISANA. Where are you located?

DIRK. Bukavu.

DR. KRISANA. Bukavu?

GEBBERS. (*Has been listening to the conversation*) Bukavu.

DIRK. Bukavu.

GEBBERS. Bukavu.

DR. KRISANA. Bukavu?

DIRK. (*Pause*) Yes.

DR. KRISANA. And where is Bukavu?

DIRK. (*Laughs*) In the Democratic Republic of Congo.

DR. KRISANA. Oh my! (*She laughs.*) I must have angels watching over me.

DIRK. Excuse me? (*Gebbers tugs at Dirk to get his attention and Dirk loses the phone connection.*)

DR. KRISANA. Nothing, nothing. I was just talking to myself. Hello? Hello?

Fade to black.

Sound: Congolese music starts.

SCENE 19. ARRIVAL (IN CONGO)

Sound: The sound of a plane landing, with music underneath. Then music fades out and we hear only the plane.

Projection: Montage of pictures from the Democratic Republic of Congo, set to music. Text "October, 2002. Democratic Republic of Congo". Text rises off the screen.

Several arriving passengers cross the stage. Dr. Krisana enters. Dirk is holding a sign that says "Dr. Kraisintu." Some arriving tourists ask Dirk where the bathroom is. Eventually Dirk sees Dr. Krisana. The following conversation is shouted over the sounds of the plane, which slowly cross-fade to jungle sounds.

DIRK. Dr. Kraisintu? Dr. Kraisintu?

DR. KRISANA. Yes! Please, call me Krisana.

DIRK. Krisana. Welcome to Africa! I am Dirk Gebbers. Horst Gebbers is my father. We spoke on the phone.

DR. KRISANA. Yes, yes, of course!

DIRK. Let me help you with that (*takes her bag*). Are you hungry? Do you want something to eat? It's going to be a long drive.

DR. KRISANA. Thank you. But no thanks.

DIRK. The car is not far from here.

DR. KRISANA. How far are we from the quinine factory?

DIRK. From Pharmakina? It's about a six-hour drive.

DR. KRISANA. How long has your factory been there?

DIRK. It was established in 1942. My father bought it in 1999.

Dirk and Dr. Krisana freeze, then begin a very slow 360° turnaround. As they turn around, the scene is reset. Trees are brought on and set all over the stage. The airplane sounds cross-fade to jungle sounds. Then Dr. Krisana and Dirk begin talking as they walk through the cinchona grove.

DR. KRISANA. The forest is beautiful.

DIRK. Our plantation extends over nearly four thousand acres. Pharmakina produces over 75 percent of the world's quinine.

DR. KRISANA. I did not know that.

DIRK. No reason you should.

DR. KRISANA. But I previously worked on several formulations with quinine, for treatment of malaria, of course. I had no idea that the world supply of quinine was so dependent on one company.

DIRK. Well, it wasn't always so. Quinine is harvested from the cinchona tree. There used to be major producers in both Peru and Indonesia. In Indonesia, the cinchona trees were destroyed by a fungal infection. In Peru, communist insurgents made it too dangerous to harvest it.

DR. KRISANA. But your trees have not been infected?

DIRK. Thank goodness, no. I have developed several new varieties of the cinchona, one of which is resistant to the Indonesian fungus.

Sound: Jungle cross fades to a quieter jungle with sounds of a stream.

SCENE 20. AT PHARMAKINA

Projection: Text "PHARMAKINA" over a panoramic photo of cinchona tree plantation.

Dr. Krisana and Dirk come forward out of the cinchona grove. Horst Gebbers enters from the forest.

GEBBERS. (*Speaking in German to someone offstage*). Der noerdliche Teil des Guts muss gewaessert werden! (*Translation: The northern part of the plantation needs water.*)

DIRK. Ah, and here is my father. Father, this is Dr. Kraisintu.

GEBBERS. (*He is very excited. He shakes her hand and says welcome twice in German*). Willkommen! Willkommen!

DR. KRISANA. Your cinchona grove is very beautiful.

GEBBERS. Danke! Danke! Willkommen! Sie muessen irgendwann auch mal unsere Gorillas sehen! (*Translation: Thank you! Thank you! Welcome! You must also see our gorillas sometime!*)

DIRK. (*Laughs at his father*) My father says thank you. Um, he also says we should show you the lowland gorillas at some point.

DR. KRISANA. Gorillas?

DIRK. Yes. There are only about eight hundred left in all of Africa. A small tribe lives here in our cinchona grove. Dr. Kraisintu, let's go inside the house. (*He calls offstage*) Mango!

GEBBERS. Mango!

They enter the house. Mango enters and waits.

DIRK. Please sit and rest a while after your long trip.

DR. KRISANA. I'm not tired. (*She sits.*)

DIRK. I'll get Mango to bring some tea. Mango, chai. (*Mango exits.*)

GEBBERS. (*To Dirk*) Erzaehl ihr von unserem Plan, erzaehl's ihr!, erzahel's ihr! (*Translation: Tell her our plan. Tell her! Tell her!*)

DIRK. (*To Gebbers*) Ja, ja, papa. (*To Dr. Krisana*) My father is very keen on your success with HIV treatments in Thailand. He would like you to help us build a small facility here, to produce HIV drugs for our workers. The problem is we cannot keep workers for the quinine production. They keep dying of AIDS.

DR. KRISANA. Only for your workers? You could do that in a kitchen, once you have a source for the drugs themselves. You then combine them into pills with my method. But why don't you make antiretrovirals for general use in the population?

DIRK. There are nearly a million people with AIDS in the DRC alone. Over 20 million in all of Africa. This is where the AIDS epidemic started.

DR. KRISANA. And so why can't it end here?

Mango returns and serves tea.

DIRK. We can't possibly make enough, even for the DRC alone.

DR. KRISANA. You have to start somewhere.

GEBBERS. (*To Dirk*) Was hat sie gesagt? (*Translation: What is she saying?*)

DIRK. Sie will viel davon herstellen. Sie will geng fuer die ganze Bevoelkerung herstellen! (*Translation: She wants to make a lot. She wants to make enough for the general population.*)

GEBBERS. Das verstehe ich nicht. (*Translation: I don't understand.*)

DIRK. Sie will eine ganz neue Fabrik aufmachen! (*Translation: She wants to make a whole new factory!*)

GEBBERS. Ja? (*Translation: Yes?*)

DIRK. Ja.

GEBBERS. Ja, ja, das ist toll. Grossartig. Phantastisch. Wunderbar. (*Translation: Yes, yes, this is great. Marvelous! Fantastic! Wonderful!*)

DIRK. (*To Dr. Krisana*) I think my father likes your idea of large-scale production.

DR. KRISANA. Excellent. Then let's get started.

DIRK. Please, Dr. Kraisintu, you must be very tired.

DR. KRISANA. I am not tired. (*She begins to take items out of a small purse and place them on a table.*) I have brought stavudine, lamivudine, and nevirapine. I have already prepared them and mixed them in the correct proportions. (*She holds up a small tube of powder.*) I also have a small hand press (*She takes this out, too, and holds it up for them to see.*). You would, of course, need a real pill press, but it is easy to demonstrate the process with this.

She puts some powder in the press and then begins to push the press together.

GEBBERS. (*Indicates that he would like to help*) Bitte. Bitte. (*Translation: Please, please.*)

Dr. Krisana gives the press to him. Gebbers pushes on the press with much grunting, then hands it back to Dr. Krisana. She opens it and takes out the pill and shows it to Gebbers and Dirk.

GEBBERS. Wunderbar! (*Joking about the size of the pill*) Un horsen pillen!

DIRK. Well, that seems quite simple, except for the grunting.

DR. KRISANA. It took several years to achieve such simplicity.

DIRK. (*Laughs*) You're talking to someone who breeds trees.

DR. KRISANA. Then I think you can appreciate—

Suddenly a bomb explodes, not far away. Dr. Krisana jumps and is quite shaken, but the others just turn to face the direction where the explosion came from. Optional: A few soldiers run across the stage, but they are not part of the immediate scene. They are somewhere else, not too far away, in the jungle.

DIRK. They have limited access to explosives or grenades. (*To Mango*) Mango? (*He motions to Mango to go check on the situation. Mango exits.*) Usually it is an isolated incident.

DR. KRISANA. Usually what is an isolated incident? What are you talking about?

DIRK. The war, of course.

DR. KRISANA. What war?

GEBBERS. (*To Dirk*) Sie hat nichts vom Krieg gehoert? (*Translation: She does not know about the war?*)

DIRK. *(To Gebbers)* Wie kann sie nichts vom Krieg gehoert haben? *(Translation: How can she not know about the war?)* *(To Dr. Krisana)* You didn't know there was a war here?

DR. KRISANA. No.

Sound: Gunfire, somewhat in the distance.

DIRK. The Second Congolese War. Some people call it the African World War because so many other countries are involved. I'm sorry, I thought the whole world knew.

DR. KRISANA. I only knew that you needed antiretrovirals.

DIRK. I'm so sorry. It never occurred to me as something that needed to be mentioned explicitly. Part of the problem is that our cinchona plantation actually crosses two borders into both Rwanda and Burundi.

GEBBERS. Burundi.

DR. KRISANA. And does the war threaten the factory?

DIRK. I'm afraid so. There are frequent evacuations. We are not a target, but sometimes the soldiers of one country or another cross through. A few months ago Rwandan troops marched through Bukavu, and the bastards raped more than fifteen thousand women in one weekend.

Mango re-enters.

DIRK. Mango?

MANGO. *(To Dirk, in Swahili)* Wamechelewa kwa siku moja pengine zaidi. *(Translation: They are very far away now.)*

DIRK. Mango says the solders we heard are gone. *(To Mango, in Swahili)* Utamsaida Daktari Kraisintu kwa lolote analohitaji. *(Translation: You will assist Dr. Kraisintu with whatever she needs.)* *(To Dr. Krisana)* Mango will be your cook and your personal assistant during your stay here.

DR. KRISANA. *(Going up to him)* Hello, Mango. I am Krisana.

MANGO. Krisana. Hujambo, Krisana. (*Translation: Hello, Krisana.*)

DIRK. Mango will also coordinate your security.

DR. KRISANA. Security?

DIRK. Yes, nothing elaborate. We just need to make sure we have a reliable guard each night for the guest house. Some of them have a tendency to fall asleep.

DR. KRISANA. I see.

DIRK. Come, let me show you the guest house.

They exit. Lights fade.

Sound: Cross-fade stream to jungle night sounds with occasional shots in the distance.

SCENE 21. SOLDIER ENCOUNTER

Sound: Jungle sounds swell.

> *It is early evening. Mango enters. He is carrying a rifle. He also has a pistol in his pocket or shoved into a belt. He brings a stool with him and perhaps something to occupy his time. He lays the rifle on the ground. After a short while we hear soft talking and laughter as some soldiers approach. Mango calmly picks up his rifle and stands. Several soldiers cross the stage. Several are carrying AK-47s. One is carrying a machete. One is barefoot. They do not see Mango and he does not see them—he only hears them. The soldiers cross directly past Mango on stage, but "in reality" they are perhaps 50–100 meters away from him. The soldiers converse mostly in Swahili, and a little bit of French. After the soldiers pass, Yosef enters.*

SOLDIER 1. Bado kitambo gani kabla hatujafika? (*Translation: How much longer till we are there?*)

SOLDIER 2. Sijui. (*Translation: I don't know.*)

SOLDIER 3. Miguu yangu inauma. (*Translation: My feet hurt.*)

SOLDIER 2. (*Laughs*) Usingaliuza viatu vyako. (*Translation: You should not have sold your shoes.*)

SOLDIER 4. Nimebakiza riasi kumi tu. (*Translation: I only have ten bullets left.*)

SOLDIER 5. Ninaichukia vita hii. (*Translation: I hate this war.*)

SOLDIER 1. Miti hii ni mizuri. (*Translation: These trees are beautiful.*)

SOLDIER 2. Pahali hapa ni pazuri. (*Translation: This place is beautiful.*)

> *The soldiers exit as Yosef enters.*

MANGO. (*He speaks first in Swahili, then repeats the line in English.*) Yosef? Ni wewe huyo Kaka? Yosef? Is that you, my brother?

YOSEF. (*He also speaks first in Swahili, then repeats it in English.*) Sht! Kelele, mjinga we! Lala tu! Shh! Be quiet, fool. Go back to sleep.

MANGO. Yosef, will there be fighting tonight?

YOSEF. Not tonight, my brother. Tonight we are only traveling through your trees. There will be no killing tonight. Who is your visitor?

MANGO. The lady?

YOSEF. Yes.

MANGO. She says she has come to make drugs to cure the slim disease.

YOSEF. You mean the HIV?

MANGO. Yes.

YOSEF. Then for sure, that is a good thing. Certainment, c'est bon.

MANGO. Yosef?

YOSEF. Yes?

MANGO. Tell me, have you seen our mother? How is she?

YOSEF. Our mother? She is dead this past month. Elle est morte.

Pause. Mango begins to quietly weep.

YOSEF. I must go. (*He starts to walk away*). Keep your lady safe, my brother. (*He exits.*)

After a moment, Dr. Krisana enters.

DR. KRISANA. Hello? Who is there? Oh, Mango, it's you. Were those soldiers that just came through the compound here? (*She looks off in the direction the soldiers went, then turns back to Mango.*) Mango. You're crying. Why are you crying?

MANGO. Amefariki mwezi jana. (*Translation: My mother has died.*)

DR. KRISANA. (*She puts her arm around Mango. He hugs her back.*) I'm sorry. I don't understand Swahili. Mango, I'm sorry that I don't know why you're crying. Perhaps something with the soldiers? The war?

MANGO. Soldiers. War. Oui.

DR. KRISANA. (*Pause*) Well, I must get some sleep now. I'm sorry, but I've been traveling for a long time. (*She pantomimes sleeping.*) Sleep. I'm going to sleep.

MANGO. Lala.

DR. KRISANA. Lala? Is that Swahili? Lala?

MANGO. Swahili.

DR. KRISANA. Lala. (*She laughs.*)

>   *There is a gunshot nearby. Both of them react.*

DR. KRISANA. You have two guns. May I have that pistol?

MANGO. (*He slowly hands her the pistol.*) Bundoki.

DR. KRISANA. Bundoki. Gun?

MANGO. Gun.

DR. KRISANA. Goodnight, Mango. (*She exits with the gun.*)

MANGO. Bon soir, madame.

Fade to black.

Sound: Music up, playing throughout the next scene.

SCENE 22. FINALE (SHADOW PLAY)

Sound: Music continues through the entire scene.

Projection: Digital scenery, clouds. The screen is cut into two parts: one for Dr. Krisana, one for Tido. The two halves are different colors.

Dr. Krisana is sitting at a table, just finishing her dinner. During the following conversation between Dr. Krisana and Tido, they start by speaking their email correspondence essentially to the audience. Slowly, their correspondence becomes more of a conversation.

DR. KRISANA. Oh, Tido. I could certainly use your help now. They want a factory here, but all they have is a war and an open field. This land, this country, is beautiful, but I've never seen so much death. We visited the main hospital in Bukavu. It's so crowded that they have two people in each bed, with their heads at opposite ends. Between AIDS, malaria, and the war, they live with death here like it's a member of the family. (*Pause*) Tido, not a single person has said the word "profit" or "patent" to me since my arrival. Tido, my friend, I hope you are well.

TIDO. (*He enters from the other side of the stage and sits at a desk and types on a laptop computer.*) Dear Krisana, it's wonderful to hear from you. Achara says it is sometimes difficult for you to email from Africa. Things are going well here with your formulations. Doctors Without Borders is buying over twenty thousand doses a day now, and the GPO is talking about scaling up manufacture again. They are selling to both Laos and Cambodia now. We miss you here.

DR. KRISANA. I'm not coming back to Thailand, Tido. This is where I am supposed to be. There is so much need here, and I can help fill it. I'm staying here.

TIDO. (*Speaking toward her, not typing*) Achara misses you. She says she thinks you're completely crazy. She says to tell you to get some sleep. And your family says the same.

DR. KRISANA. Well, okay, I will come to visit my family, of course. Samui Island is the source of my strength. It is the heart of my world. But my work there, in Thailand, is done. My work is here now. It's so clear. This is a new beginning for me.

TIDO. Perhaps you have heard, but Brighton Miles has backed down from our lawsuit and decided to donate the Thai patent rights for ddI to the people of Thailand. After so long! The GPO has begun to look into manufacture of antiretrovirals with ddI in them again—I think they are going back to your original formulations. We waited years for a resolution of this case, and then they simply turn and walk away. They are cowards.

DR. KRISANA. All bullies are cowards in the end. These things are an ocean away from me now. No U.S. patents are recognized here. There are no TRIPs agreements here. At least, not yet. Tido! I'm going to manufacture antiretrovirals in the jungles of Africa!

Sound: BBC newscast.

Projection: BBC newscast is broadcast onscreen, replacing the shadow-play imagery, but with Dr. Krisana and Tido's shadows still visible.

SELENA SCOTT. Good evening, I'm Selena Scott and this is the BBC World Service for July 16, 2005. A small pharmaceutical firm in the Democratic Republic of Congo this week became the first company on the African continent to initiate large-scale manufacture of treatments for HIV/AIDS. While donations have steadily risen in recent years, local manufacture of needed drugs in Africa remains almost non-existent. (*Volume slowly fades back into music.*) Scientists at the Pharmakina corporation have spent nearly

81

two and one-half years preparing for their opening production run, and will produce a triple-drug HIV cocktail (*she repeats the word "cocktail" several times, as though there is a glitch in the video, and/or from different camera angles*) they are calling Afri-VIR. Such single-pill formulations are rapidly becoming a worldwide standard. (*BBC sound fades, leaving only music*).

Projection: BBC cross-fades back to shadow-play imagery (clouds).

TIDO. (*Raising a glass*) Never give up, Krisana. Never give up.
Dr. Krisana responds by raising her glass. Music swells. Grandmother enters in shadow play and stands behind Dr. Krisana, placing her hand on her shoulder.

Fade to black.

THE END